Mary Johnson

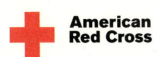 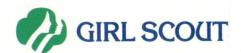 

SMALL CRAFT
SAFETY

The American Red Cross Small Craft Safety program
is endorsed by:

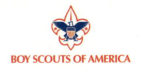

BOY SCOUTS OF AMERICA

When in danger in a kayak or canoe:
wave paddle for attention

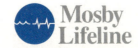

St. Louis Baltimore Boston Carlsbad Chicago Naples New York Philadelphia Portland
London Madrid Mexico City Singapore Sydney Tokyo Toronto Wiesbaden

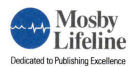

**A Times Mirror
Company**

Copyright © 1998 by The American National Red Cross

All rights reserved. No part of this publication may be reproduced, stored in a retrieval system, or transmitted in any form or by any means, electronic, mechanical, photocopying, recording, or otherwise, without prior written permission from the publisher.

This participant's manual is an integral part of American Red Cross training. By itself, it does not constitute complete and comprehensive training.

The emergency care procedures outlined in this book reflect the standard of knowledge and accepted emergency practices in the United States at the time this book was published. It is the reader's responsibility to stay informed of changes in the emergency care procedures.

Printed in the United States of America

Composition by Accu-Color
Printing/Binding by The Banta Book Group

Mosby Lifeline
Mosby–Year Book, Inc.
11830 Westline Industrial Drive
St. Louis, MO 63146

Library of Congress Cataloging-in-Publication Data

Small craft safety / American Red Cross.
      p.   cm.
   Includes bibliographical references and index.
   ISBN 0-8151-7956-1
   1. Boats and boating—Safety measures.   I. American Red Cross.
VK200.S53   1997
797.1'028'9—dc21   97-37607
                                                        CIP

97 98 99 00 01 / 9 8 7 6 5 4 3 2 1

Acknowledgments

This workbook was developed through the combined effort of the American Red Cross, the American Camping Association, and the Girl Scouts of the USA. Without the commitment to excellence of the paid and volunteer staff from these organizations, this workbook could not have been created.

The Health and Safety Services Water Safety Project Development Team at American Red Cross national headquarters responsible for designing and writing this participant's workbook include the following: Mike Espino, Senior Associate, Project Team Leader; Rhonda Starr, Project Manager; Don K. Vardell, MS, Senior Associate; Tab Bates, NREMT-B; Stephen Bartos, MBS; Stephen Lynch, Jose Salazar, and Connie Tippett, Associates, Educational Development; Ann Dioda, Associate, Program and Customer Support; Marietta Damond, Senior Associate, Program Evaluation; and Jane Moore, Specialist. Administrative support for the project was provided by Vivian Mills.

The following American Camping Association personnel provided guidance and review: Margery M. Scanlin, Ed.D., Division Director; Karen D. Sivia, Director, Field Service; and Greg Shute, The Chewonki Foundation, Wiscasset, Maine.

The following Girl Scouts of the USA staff provided guidance and review: Donna L. Nye, Membership and Program Consultant; Carolyn L. Kennedy, Director of Special Projects, Membership and Program; and Verna Simpkins, Director of Membership and Program Services, Membership and Program.

The following American Red Cross national headquarters Health and Safety Services staff provided guidance and review: Susan M. Livingstone, Vice President, Health and Safety Services; Ferris D. Kaplan, Director, Business Development and Marketing; Anthony Gallagher, Manager, Program Evaluation; Earl Harbert, Manager, Contract and Financial Management; Dana Jessen, Manager, Program and Customer Support; Linwood Tucker, Associate, Risk Management; and Martin Sarsfield, Analyst, Risk Management.

The Mosby Lifeline Editorial and Production Team included: Claire Merrick, Editor-in-Chief; Valerie Stewart, Senior Marketing Manager; Lisa Benson, Editorial Project Supervisor; Shannon Canty, and Nadine Steffan, Project Supervisors; Doug Bruce, Director, Lifeline EDP; and Eric Duchinsky, Editor.

Special thanks go to: Tim McQuade, Erie Community College, Buffalo, New York, writer; Tom Lochhaas, Developmental Editor; Vincent Knaus, Photographer; Craig Reinertson, Manager, AV Studio; and Richard Even, Christopher Johnson, and Steve Menicks, video producers/directors, American Red Cross; Doug Braswell, REI, Bailey's Crossroads, VA.

Guidance and review were also provided by members of the Water Safety Project Ad Hoc group:

Byron F. Andrews, III, Sterling Volunteer Rescue Squad, Sterling, Virginia

Mary Essert, Essert Associates, Inc., El Cerrito, California

Jerry Huey, American Red Cross—Southeastern Michigan Chapter, Detroit, Michigan

Lt. Patrick J. Marston, Alabama Marine Police, Mobile, Alabama

Toni Marie O'Donnell, City of Los Angeles, Los Angeles, California

Laura J. Slane, YMCA of USA, Chicago, Illinois

Wm. E. Staiger, Ohio Department of Natural Resources, Division of Watercraft, Akron, Ohio

External review was provided by the following individuals:

Alex Antoniou, Ph. D., Rutgers University, Piscataway, New Jersey

Julian K. "Duke" Brown, M.Ed., SCEMT-I, Horry County Beach Safety—HCPD, Conway, South Carolina

Lt. Ray Cranston, Farmington Hills Police Department, Farmington Hills, Michigan

Dean W. Dimke, American Red Cross in Delaware, Wilmington, Delaware

Acknowledgments

Joan Drnek, Lake Erie Girl Scout Council, Cleveland, Ohio

Lynn L. Etnier, B.S., Camp We-Ha-Kee, Winter, Wisconsin

Ginny Long, United States Sailing Association, Portsmouth, Rhode Island

Jo Mogle, United States Sailing Association, Portsmouth, Rhode Island

Lawrence D. Newell, Ed.D., NREMT-P, NAI Consultants, Ashburn, Virginia

James S. O'Connor, M.S., Metropolitan Dade County, Miami, Florida

Slim Ray, Ashville, North Carolina

H. Bradford Rounds, American Red Cross Portland Chapter, Portland, Maine

Daniel R. Ruth, Boy Scouts of America, Irving, Texas

Jim Segerstrom, Rescue III International, Sonora, California

David S. Smith, Smith Aquatic Safety Services, Charlevoi, Michigan

Diane Tyrrell, Girl Scout Council of Colonial Coast, Chesapeake, Virginia

Susan K. Wagner, American Red Cross Central Panhandle Chapter, Panama City, Florida

Charlie Walbridge, American Canoe Association, Blue Belle, Pennsylvania

Phyllis Woestemeyer, M.A., MICP, Piscataway Township Public Schools, Piscataway, New Jersey

The following original materials were produced under a grant funded by the Aquatic Resources (Wallop/Breaux) Trust Fund, administered by the U.S. Coast Guard. Reprinted by permission of the American Camping Association, Martinsville, IN and the U.S. Coast Guard, Washington, DC.

- Appendix B
- Selected glossary terms

How to Use This Workbook

This workbook is designed to help you learn and understand the material it presents. It includes the following features:

Objectives

At the beginning of each chapter is a list of objectives that describe what you should know and be able to do after reading the chapter and participating in class activities. Read these objectives carefully and refer back to them from time to time as you read the chapter.

Key Terms

At the beginning of each chapter is a list of defined key terms that you need to know to understand chapter content. In the chapter, key terms are printed in bold italics the first time they are defined or explained.

Sidebars

Feature articles called sidebars enhance the information in the main body of the text. They appear in most chapters and present a variety of information to enhance the main body of the text. You will not be tested on any information presented in these sidebars as part of the American Red Cross course completion requirements.

Learning Activities

Learning activities appear in each of the craft chapters (Chapters 4-7) and at the end of each chapter. They are designed to help you understand and remember the material presented in the chapter. Answering these questions after you have read the chapter will help you evaluate your progress and prepare for the final written examination. Many of the multiple choice questions have more than one correct answer. Discuss any questions with which you have difficulty with your instructor.

Appendixes

Appendixes are located at the end of this textbook and provide additional information on topics that boaters will find useful.

Glossary

The glossary includes definitions of all key terms and of other words in the text that may be unfamiliar. All glossary terms appear in the textbook in bold type the first time they are used or explained.

Contents

CHAPTER 1 *Small Craft Safety* 1

Introduction 2
Water Safety Guidelines 2
Open-Water Environments 2
   Lakes and Ponds 2
   Rivers and Streams 3
   The Ocean 3
Types of Small Craft 3
   The Canoe 3
   The Kayak 4
   The Sailboat 4
   The Rowboat 4
Preventing Small Craft Accidents,
Injuries, and Fatalities 4
   Alcohol and Water Do Not Mix 5
   Life Jackets 5
   Preventing Capsizes and Falls Overboard 6
   Preventing Collisions 7
Legal Requirements 7
   Small Craft Registration 7
   Personal Flotation Devices (PFDs) 8
   Sound Devices 8
   Craft Capacity 8
   Navigation Lights 8
   Visual Distress Signals 8
   Accident Reporting 8
Summary 8
Learning Activities 9

CHAPTER 2 *Trip Planning, Supervision,*
and Emergency Preparation 11

Introduction 12
Small Craft Trip Planning 12
   Selecting a Leader 12
   Responsibilities and Legal Considerations 12
   Selecting the Locale and Route 12
   Checking the Weather Conditions 12
   Checking the Water Conditions 13
   Choosing the Appropriate Equipment 14
   Safety Equipment 14
   Checking the Craft and Equipment 14
   Choosing the Appropriate Clothing 15

Small Craft Supervision 15
   Communication 15
   Leader-to-Participant Ratios 15
   Leader Location 15
Emergency Preparation 15
   Emergency Action Plan 16
   After an Emergency 17
Summary 19
Learning Activities 19

CHAPTER 3 *Basic Water Rescue* 22

Introduction 23
Self-Rescue 23
   Survival Floating 23
   Self-Rescue When Clothed 23
   Self-Rescue When Wearing a Life Jacket 25
Rescuing Others 26
   Recognizing Aquatic Emergencies 26
   Rescue Guidelines 27
   Reaching Assist with Equipment 27
   Reaching Assist without Equipment 28
   Throwing Assist 28
   Wading Assist with Equipment 30
   Removal from the Water 30
Emergency Care 31
   Head, Neck, and Back Injury 31
   Hypothermia 32
   Seizures 34
   Unconscious Victim 34
   Emergency Care 34
Summary 35
Learning Activities 35

CHAPTER 4 *Canoeing Safety* 38

Introduction 39
The Canoe 39
   Learning Activity 39
Canoeing Safety 39
   Preventing Canoe Capsizes, Falls Overboard,
      and Collisions 40
   Guidelines for Safe Canoeing 40
Supervision and Communication 40

v

Canoeing Emergencies 40
    Rescue Priorities 40
    Canoeing Emergencies in Flat Water 40
Summary 44
Learning Activities 44

CHAPTER 5 *Kayaking Safety* 46

Introduction 47
The Kayak 47
    Learning Activity 47
Kayaking Safety 47
    Guidelines for Safe Kayaking 48
Supervision and Communication 48
Kayaking Emergencies 48
    Rescue Priorities 48
    Kayaking Emergencies in Flat Water 48
Summary 51
Learning Activities 51

CHAPTER 6 *Sailing Safety* 53

Introduction 54
The Sailboat 54
    Learning Activity 54
Sailing Safety 54
    Preventing Sailing Accidents, Injuries, and Fatalities 54
Supervision and Communication 57
Sailing Emergencies 58
    Rescue Priorities 58
    Self-Rescue after Sailboat Capsize 58
    Overboard Recovery 59
Summary 60
Learning Activities 60

CHAPTER 7 *Rowing Safety* 62

Introduction 63
The Rowboat 63
    Learning Activity 63
Rowing Safety 63
    Preventing Rowing Accidents, Injuries, and Fatalities 63

Rowing Emergencies 64
    Rescue Priorities 64
    Self-Rescue 64
    Rescuing Others from the Water 64
Summary 67
Learning Activities 67

CHAPTER 8 *Moving-Water Safety— Canoeing and Kayaking* 69

Introduction 70
Moving-Water Safety 70
    Guidelines for Moving-Water Safety 70
Supervision and Communication on Moving Water 70
Moving-Water Emergencies 71
    Self-Rescue in Moving Water 71
    Rescuing Others in Moving Water 74
Summary 76
Learning Activities 76

GLOSSARY 79

LEARNING ACTIVITY ANSWERS 82

APPENDIXES

APPENDIX A *River Hazards* 86

APPENDIX B *The International Scale of River Difficulty* 88

APPENDIX C *Small Craft/Water Safety Organizations and Resources* 89

APPENDIX D *Float Plan* 91

APPENDIX E *Accident Report Form* 92

APPENDIX F *State Boating Law Administrators* 95

REFERENCES 99

INDEX 100

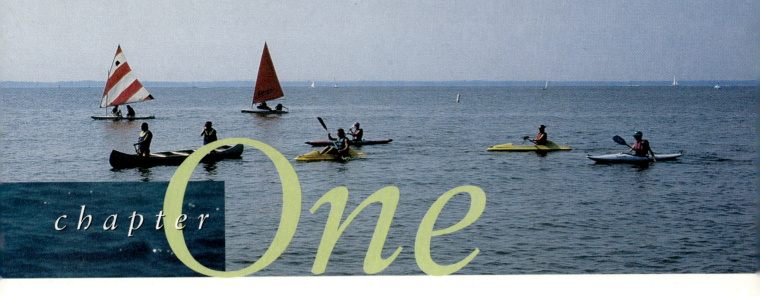

chapter One

Small Craft Safety

OBJECTIVES

After reading this chapter you should be able to—
1. List water safety guidelines for activities in, on, or around the water.
2. Identify different types of open-water environments and their potential hazards.
3. Identify the types of small craft.
4. Explain the primary causes of boating accidents, injuries, and fatalities.
5. Explain the importance of wearing a life jacket when boating.
6. Describe how to prevent small craft accidents, injuries, and fatalities.
7. Identify and explain the rules of the road.
8. List and explain the legal requirements that apply to small craft.
9. Define the key terms for this chapter.

KEY TERMS

Canoe: A light, slender boat with a pointed bow and pointed or square stern, generally propelled by single-blade paddles.
Capsize: To turn a craft upside down in the water.
Collision: A craft crashing into another craft or object.
Drowning: Death by suffocation underwater.
Fall overboard: To unintentionally fall out of a craft into the water.
Kayak: A decked boat with pointed ends and a cockpit, propelled by a double-blade paddle.
Life jacket: A type of personal flotation device (PFD) that can be worn.

Open water: Natural bodies of water, such as lakes, ponds, rivers, streams, and the ocean.
Personal Flotation Device (PFD): Life jacket, buoyancy vest, wearable flotation aid, throwable flotation aid, deck suit, work vest, sailboarding vest, or hybrid inflatable flotation aid.
Rowboat: A small, open boat propelled by oars.
Rules of the Road: Navigation rules indicating right-of-way among boats to prevent collisions.
Sailboat: A boat with one or more sails, powered by wind.
Trim: The balance of a craft from front to back.

INTRODUCTION

Boating activity has increased rapidly in recent years. Many types of water craft are used for recreation, business, sport, and transportation. The United States Coast Guard estimates that there are about 20 million recreational boats in the United States.

The term *small craft* is used to describe several different types of small boats. In this workbook, small craft are nonmotorized recreational water craft. The American Red Cross Small Craft Safety course and workbook focus on **canoes, kayaks,** small **sailboats,** and **rowboats.**

Boating can be safe and enjoyable when everyone is careful. Unfortunately emergencies still occur. This workbook will help you to recognize, prevent, and respond to small craft emergencies. You will learn about small craft trip planning, supervision, and emergency preparation. You will also learn how to protect yourself while assisting others.

The information in this workbook is intended for—

- Camp personnel, trip leaders, and small craft instructors.
- Clubs and organizations that engage in small craft activities, such as the Girl Scouts of the USA, Boy Scouts of America, and Boy's and Girl's Clubs of America.
- Anyone involved in small craft activities for recreation, sport, work, or just for fun.

The information in this workbook is *not* intended to—

- Teach small craft operational skills, such as paddling, rowing, or sailing.
- Provide information and skills needed to become or qualify as a lifeguard.

For information on these types of specialized training, contact your local Red Cross.

WATER SAFETY GUIDELINES

Everyone should follow safety guidelines when in, on, or around the water. These guidelines are especially important if you are leading or instructing others in a small craft activity or responding to a small craft emergency. The following are general water safety guidelines:

- Learn to swim.
- Learn boating, CPR, and first aid skills.
  - Contact your local Red Cross for information about swimming, first aid, and CPR courses.
  - Check with your local Red Cross, the U.S. Coast Guard, state boating officials, and other organizations about boating courses. (See Appendix C for a list of boating and other water safety organizations.)
- Always supervise children in, on, or around the water.
- Do not drink alcohol while swimming or boating.
- Know what to do in case of a small craft emergency.
- Do not attempt a swimming rescue unless you have specialized training and proper equipment. Remember, you can help a victim only if you stay safe yourself.
- Wear a U.S. Coast Guard-approved *life jacket* when around water or when boating.
- Be aware of potential water hazards.
- Pay attention to local weather conditions and forecasts.
- Know how to prevent accidents, recognize hazards, and care for injuries.

OPEN-WATER ENVIRONMENTS

Knowing the different types of open-water environments and their potential hazards is an important part of water safety. **Open water** has unique hazards and conditions that may change from hour to hour due to weather, tides, or currents. Check for hazards before allowing others to enter the water or go boating. The following sections describe different types of open-water environments and their possible hazards.

Lakes and Ponds

The water in lakes and ponds can be **murky** making it difficult to see below the surface. Murky conditions make it more difficult to see or rescue a submerged victim (Fig. 1-1). You may not be able to see pieces of debris and obstructions or determine the depth of the water. Serious injury or death can result from diving into water of unknown depth. Weeds and plant life may make it hard to see the bottom or may entangle swimmers. Rocks just below the surface may create obstacles for boats. Like other open-water environments, conditions in lakes and ponds can change rapidly because of weather or currents.

Figure 1-1

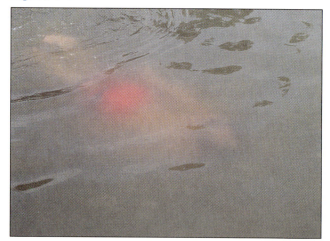

CHAPTER 1 *Small Craft Safety* 3

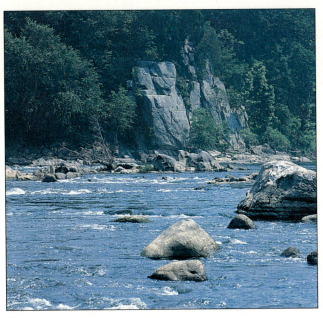

Figure 1-2

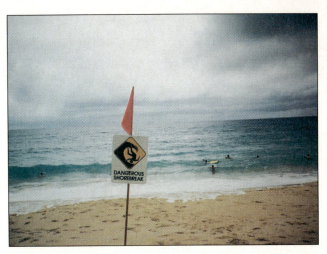

Figure 1-3

Rivers and Streams

Heavy rainfall and melting snow have dramatic effects on rivers. When flooding occurs, slow-moving water can quickly become a raging current. River water can be dangerously cold, especially during the winter and spring months, and in colder parts of the country. Rivers and streams often have rocks, debris, **low-head dams, hydraulics,** steep drops, dams, falls, **strainers,** and other hazardous obstacles (Fig. 1-2). (See Chapter 8 for more information on river hazards.)

River currents can be unpredictable and fast moving. The current's direction may change abruptly because of changes in the river bottom. The current may be stronger in some areas than in others, and usually flows faster in shallow areas than in deep areas.

When currents are slow and **waves** are fairly calm, you generally can help a person in trouble. However, when currents are strong and water is cold, giving assistance may be difficult or impossible. In this situation, call for help immediately. (Refer to Chapter 8 for information on recognizing, preventing, and responding to emergencies in a moving-water environment.)

The Ocean

Oceans pose a number of potential hazards, including waves, currents, sandbars, and other changing conditions (Fig. 1-3). Although these conditions are often more hazardous to swimmers close to shore, boaters must also be aware of them. Strong breaking waves can potentially capsize and injure a boater entering or exiting at the shore. Dangerous currents can carry a person or boat away from shore.

TYPES OF SMALL CRAFT

Hundreds of styles of small boats are available today. Small craft have widely varying characteristics, features, and equipment. Although every boat handles differently, the same general safety guidelines apply to each. Four basic types of small craft—canoe, kayak, sailboat, and rowboat—are described below. Chapters 4 to 7 give more details on these boats and the specific safety and rescue procedures appropriate for each.

The Canoe

Canoes are popular open water craft that are used on almost all kinds of water. Canoes of different sizes and materials have been developed for different uses and water conditions (Fig. 1-4).

Figure 1-4

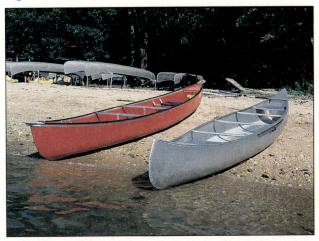

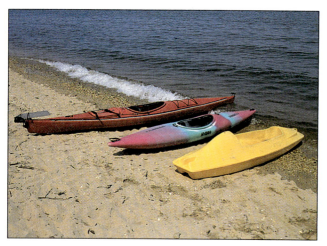

Figure 1-5

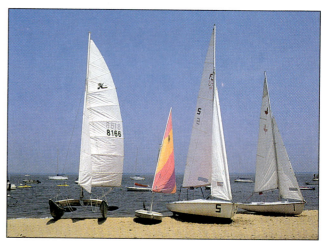

Figure 1-6

The Kayak

Kayaks are constructed from a variety of materials and come in many styles, including white-water, sit-on-top, inflatable, tandem, and sea kayaks (Fig. 1-5). Many kayaks are **decked** boats except for the paddler's opening (**cockpit**).

The Sailboat

Sailboats are powered by one or more sails. Sailboats are available in a wide variety of sizes, shapes, and designs, and have varying characteristics and purposes (Fig. 1-6).

The Rowboat

The most common type of rowboat used for recreation has a flat bottom. Flat-bottom rowboats are designed for calm waters. Like other types of small craft, there are several types of rowboats, varying from wooden skiffs to fiberglass dinghies to aluminum jonboats (Fig. 1-7).

Figure 1-7

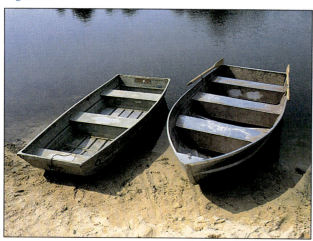

PREVENTING SMALL CRAFT ACCIDENTS, INJURIES, AND FATALITIES

Drowning is the fourth most common cause of death from unintentional injury in the United States (Fig. 1-8). Approximately 4,500 Americans drown every year. Boating activity in the United States results in thousands of accidents and

Figure 1-8

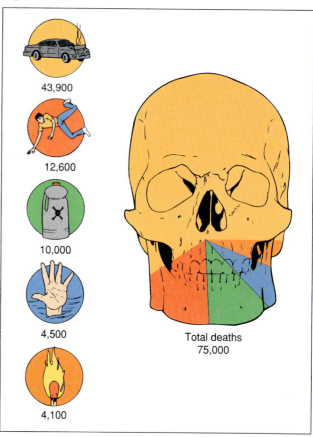

injuries, and hundreds of fatalities every year. To help reduce the number of deaths and injuries, boaters need to be educated on the fundamentals of small craft safety. Understanding the causes of small craft accidents, injuries, and fatalities can help people learn to prevent them. With proper training and adequate knowledge, many boating accidents can be avoided. Consider these facts about boating accidents and fatalities:

- Most boating accidents are caused by the operator, not by the boat or the aquatic environment.
- Most fatalities involve boats less than 16 feet long.
- Approximately 80 percent of the boating fatalities in the United States are drownings, and most of these drownings would not have occurred if the boater had been wearing a U.S. Coast Guard-approved life jacket.
- Most drownings occur when a boater unexpectedly enters the water. This happens when a boat *capsizes,* when a boater *falls overboard,* or when a *collision* occurs with another boat or object.

In addition to the hundreds of boating fatalities and thousands of serious injuries, boating accidents cause millions of dollars in property damage each year. The following sections describe how you can prevent small craft accidents, injuries, and fatalities.

Alcohol and Water Do Not Mix

Drinking alcohol in, on, or around the water is dangerous. The U.S. Coast Guard reports that more than half of boating-related drownings involve alcohol. Even a little alcohol can lead to a dangerous situation. Drinking alcohol—

- Affects balance, making it more likely that someone will fall into the water.
- Makes it harder to stay warm, even though it may initially give the illusion of warmth.
- Affects judgment and may encourage risk taking, such as diving into shallow or unknown water.
- Slows body movements and impairs vision.
- Reduces a person's boating and swimming skills.

Life Jackets

There are five approved types of *personal flotation devices* (PFDs) (Table 1-1). Types I, II, III, and V (inflatable only) are commonly referred to as life jackets.

Always wear a U.S. Coast Guard-approved life jacket when boating. The Coast Guard-approved label is attached to or printed directly on the life jacket. In addition to keeping you afloat, a life jacket will help conserve body heat and can protect you from the impact of rocks, debris, or another

TABLE 1-1

TYPE	STYLE	ILLUSTRATION	TYPICAL USE	FEATURES
I	Life jacket		Boating on offshore waters where rescue may be delayed.	May help turn an unconscious person in the water from a face-down position to a vertical, face-up position, or a slightly tipped-back position.
II	Buoyant vest		Recreational boating on inland waters where a rescue is likely to occur quickly.	May help turn an unconscious person in the water from a face-down position to a vertical, face-up position, or a slightly tipped-back position. Less buoyant than Type I life jacket.
III	Flotation vest		Paddling or sailing on inland waters where a rescue is likely to occur quickly.	May help keep a conscious person in a vertical, face-up position, or a slightly tipped-back position.
IV	Throwable device, such as buoyant cushion or ring buoy		Boating on inland waters with heavy boat traffic where help is always present.	May be thrown to a victim in an emergency. Does not take the place of wearing a life jacket or vest.
V	Special use, including hybrid inflatable PFD		Intended for specific activities, such as sailboarding.	Must be used according to directions on its label to be acceptable. A hybrid inflatable PFD must be worn to comply with legal requirements.

Illustrations from USCG Auxiliary: *Boating Safely.* Used with permission.

craft, but only if you *have it on*. Boating accidents happen quickly and unexpectedly. If an accident occurs, you will not have time to put your life jacket on, and may not even be able to find it. When supervising small craft activities, make sure everyone on board is wearing a properly fitted life jacket that is in good condition.

Choosing the right life jacket depends on the activity you are participating in and the water conditions. It should be in good condition and fit properly for your size and weight (Fig. 1-9). Never substitute a child-sized life jacket for an adult-sized life jacket or an adult-sized life jacket for a child-sized life jacket. A properly fitted life jacket should feel snug. Once you have a properly fitted life jacket, put it on and practice moving around in shallow water to get accustomed to wearing it. Check the buoyancy of the life jacket by relaxing your body and tilting your head back. The life jacket should keep your chin above water, allowing you to breathe.

Do not sit or kneel on a life jacket, such improper use can damage it. A damaged life jacket is no longer Coast Guard-approved.

Preventing Capsizes and Falls Overboard

Most boating fatalities result from capsizes or falls overboard. These accidents are more common on small craft. Most can be prevented by keeping the craft balanced and in good *trim*.

To stay balanced in a small craft—

- Do not sit on the **gunwale**.
- Keep your weight low and centered in the craft.
- When moving around in a boat, have two hands and one foot, or one hand and two feet in contact with the boat (Fig. 1-10).

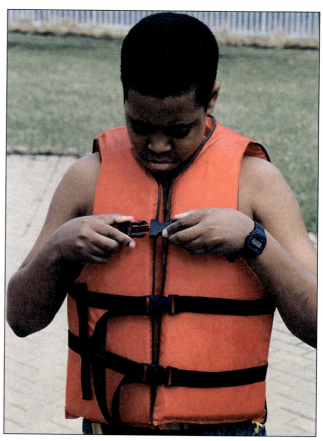

Figure 1-9

Trimming the craft means correctly balancing the craft by having the weight properly distributed between the front and the back. To trim your craft, evenly distribute the gear and passengers in the boat.

Additional causes of capsizes or falls overboard include waves, high winds, and sudden or unexpected turns. Prevent these hazards by paying attention to what you are doing, and by communicating with others around you. To avoid capsizing, steer your craft directly into large waves

Figure 1-10

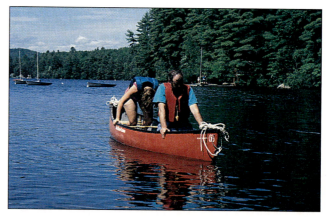

Inflatable PFDs

In April 1996 the U.S. Coast Guard adopted rules for "inflatable" PFDs. Unlike traditional "filled" PFDs, these "inflatable" PFDs consist of hollow bladders that are automatically inflated with carbon dioxide from a small canister. They can also be inflated by pulling a cord on the vest or by blowing into an inflation port.

Inflatable PFDs have been popular in other countries for years. They are lightweight and allow a person to move easily while wearing the device. These features make them a good choice for those who wear PFDs for long periods of time, such as people who work around the water.

The disadvantages of inflatable PFDs include their higher initial cost and routine maintenance of the carbon dioxide canister and triggering device. Inflatable PFDs must have a visual indicator that the carbon dioxide canister has not been discharged. Inflatable PFDs are not approved for children and are not recommended for nonswimmers.

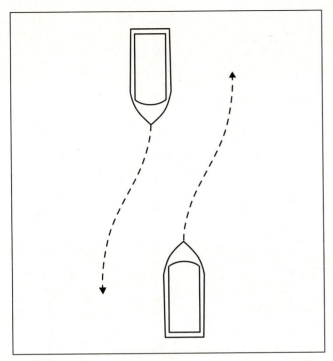

Figure 1-11

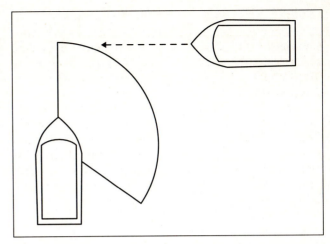

Figure 1-12

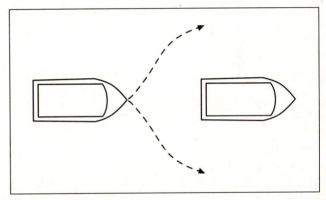

Figure 1-13

rather than letting the waves hit the craft broadside. Be sure to advise your passengers before you turn the craft. Do not go out on the water if wind or water conditions are beyond your ability, or if they are too rough for the type and size of small craft you are operating.

Preventing Collisions

Collisions with other boats or objects account for about half of all boating accidents. Collisions often result from boater carelessness or ignorance of the boating *rules of the road.* To prevent collisions, the operator of a small craft must look out for other craft and submerged objects, and must follow the rules of the road.

Rules of the Road
Whether canoeing, kayaking, sailing, or rowing, boaters should know and follow the rules of the road:

- When approaching another craft head-on, both craft keep to their right (just like cars traveling in opposite directions on a two-lane road) (Fig. 1-11).
- When crossing paths, the craft on the right has right-of-way (Fig. 1-12).
- When passing another craft from behind, the craft being overtaken has right-of-way (Fig. 1-13).
- Even if one craft has the right-of-way, both craft are responsible for avoiding a collision. Always take action to avoid a collision. Never assume that the operator of another craft knows the rules of the road.

Different rules apply when small craft meet certain types of larger craft and craft under sail. To be safe in all situations, know what rules apply for situations you are likely to encounter in your boating area. Contact the local U.S. Coast Guard office or state boating administrator in your area (Appendix F) for more information.

LEGAL REQUIREMENTS

Federal and state laws regulate water craft operation. These laws often relate to safety and, in general, protect the well-being and interests of the overall boating community. Make sure you know the federal and state laws that apply to you and your craft.

Small Craft Registration

In some states all water craft are required to be registered with the state. Other states require motorboats, sailboats, or water craft over a certain length to be registered.

Personal Flotation Devices (PFDs)

Federal law mandates that boats less than 16 feet must carry a wearable PFD for each person on board. Boats 16 feet and over must also have at least one type IV PFD aboard. Wearable PFDs must be U.S. Coast Guard-approved, readily accessible, and properly sized.

Sound Devices

Due to the dangers of fog, mist, and rain, all craft are required by federal law to have a sound device on board. Craft shorter than 39.4 feet can use a whistle, horn, or bell as a sound signal.

Craft Capacity

Small craft, like any other water craft, may not be operated over capacity. Most craft have a capacity plate that indicates the maximum weight or number of people allowed on board. If your craft does not have a capacity plate, you can calculate its maximum capacity. Multiply the length of the craft, in feet, by the **beam** (width at the widest part), and divide by 15 (fractions should be rounded down).

$$\text{Maximum \# of people} = \frac{\text{Length} \times \text{Beam}}{15}$$

Navigation Lights

Most small craft are not equipped for nighttime travel. However, federal law requires that all craft on the water between sundown and sunup, and during other periods of reduced visibility have navigation lights on board and in use. Electric torches, flashlights, or lighted lanterns with white lights are acceptable navigational lights for small craft in most states.

Visual Distress Signals

Visual distress signals are emergency devices used by craft in distress. Federal law mandates that craft operating at night carry nighttime visual distress signals, such as hand-held flares, aerial flares, or distress lights when operating on coastal waters.

Accident Reporting

If a serious boating accident or injury occurs, the proper marine law authorities must be notified, and a boating accident report must be filed in the state where the accident occurred. For a copy of the Accident Report Form see Appendix E. The U.S. Coast Guard requires that the following boating accidents be reported:

- An accident that results in death
- An accident that results in injury and requires medical attention beyond first aid
- An accident that results in property damage of $500 or more, or the complete loss of a craft

Different legal requirements apply to different types and sizes of small craft. For further information on federal and state boating laws, contact the local U.S. Coast Guard office or state boating administrator in your area (Appendix F).

SUMMARY

Boating and other water activities can be safe and enjoyable. Follow the water safety guidelines, and understand the different types of open-water environments and their potential hazards. Understand the primary causes of small craft injuries, accidents, and fatalities. Prevent small craft accidents, injuries, and fatalities by—

- Using life jackets properly.
- Preventing capsizes, falls overboard, and collisions.
- Avoiding drinking alcohol when boating.
- Knowing the rules of the road.
- Meeting legal requirements for small craft.

CHAPTER 1 *Small Craft Safety*

LEARNING ACTIVITIES

TRUE OR FALSE

Circle the correct answer.

1. You should attempt a swimming rescue if you have no training but have the proper equipment. True or False?

2. Open water refers only to the open ocean or large inland bodies of water, such as the great lakes. True or False?

3. A fast-moving section of a river with rapids is generally shallower than a section with a slow current and smooth surface. True or False?

4. When approaching another craft head-on, both craft should keep to their right. True or False?

5. When crossing paths, the craft on the right has the right-of-way. True or False?

6. The U.S. Coast Guard requires one PFD for every two people on board. True or False?

7. A whistle, horn, or bell can be used as a sounding device on a small craft. True or False?

MULTIPLE CHOICE

Circle the letter of the best answer or answers.

1. Drinking alcohol in, on, or around the water is dangerous because it—
    a. Impairs swimming skills.
    b. Impairs judgment.
    c. Reduces the ability to stay warm.
    d. Affects balance.
    e. All of the above.

2. Which of the following are correct statements about small craft accidents, injuries, and fatalities?
    a. Most fatalities involve boats less than 16 feet long.
    b. Most boating accidents are caused by the aquatic environment—not the operator.
    c. Most drownings happen when a boat capsizes, a boater falls overboard, or when a collision occurs.
    d. About 80 percent of boating fatalities are drownings, and could have been prevented if the boater were wearing a life jacket.

3. Which of the following are correct statements about life jackets and boating?
    a. Most people who drown from boating accidents are not wearing a life jacket.
    b. You do not need a life jacket if you know how to swim.
    c. Wearing a life jacket will help conserve body heat and keep you afloat.
    d. A life jacket may protect you from impact from rocks, debris, or another craft.
    e. If someone needs your assistance in the water, you both are safer if you are wearing a life jacket.
    f. You should have the life jacket close by, not on you.

4. Which of the following are the correct actions to prevent capsizes and falls overboard?
    a. Stand up in the craft.
    b. Do not sit on the gunwale.
    c. When moving around in a boat, have two hands and one foot, or one hand and two feet in contact with the boat.
    d. Put most of the passengers and gear towards the rear of the craft.
    e. Pay attention to what you are doing, and communicate with others around you.

5. Which of the following statements is NOT correct?
    a. Life jackets should always be worn when boating.
    b. A properly fitted life jacket should feel snug.
    c. Inflatable Type V life jackets can be used as seat cushions.
    d. Make sure your life jacket is U.S. Coast Guard-approved.

6. To avoid collisions while boating—
    a. Learn and follow the boating rules of the road.
    b. Register your craft with the proper authorities.
    c. Keep a proper lookout for other craft and submerged objects.
    d. a and c.

SMALL CRAFT SAFETY

FILL IN

Fill in the correct answers.

1. You want to go boating with some friends. Your craft is 14 feet long, and the beam is 5 feet. What is the maximum number of people allowed in the craft? _____

SCENARIO

1. You are taking a group of campers out on the water. The trip will be on a lake.

2. List 5 or more potential hazards found in different types of open-water environments. _____
_____
_____

a. List at least three water safety guidelines you should follow. _____
_____
_____
_____

b. What type of hazards could you expect? _____
_____

c. What advice can you give the group to avoid capsizes, falls overboard, and collisions? _____
_____
_____
_____

d. Should you and all participants be wearing life jackets? _____

e. Why or why not? _____
_____
_____

See answers to learning activities on page 82.

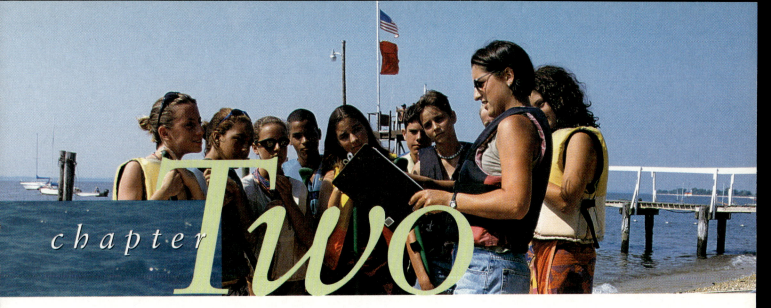

chapter Two

Trip Planning, Supervision, and Emergency Preparation

OBJECTIVES

After reading this chapter you should be able to—
1. Identify the steps in planning a safe and enjoyable small craft outing.
2. Describe the responsibilities and legal considerations for group leaders.
3. Identify what information should be included in a float plan.
4. Recognize hazardous weather conditions, and know what to do if a storm approaches.
5. Identify safety equipment and appropriate clothing for a safe trip.
6. Explain the importance of communication, leader-to-participant ratios, and leader location.
7. Discuss how to prepare for an emergency.
8. Write and develop an emergency action plan (EAP).
9. Define the key terms for this chapter.

KEY TERMS

Critical Incident Stress: The stress a person experiences during or after a highly stressful emergency.
Emergency Action Plan (EAP): A written plan detailing how members of a group are to respond in a specific type of emergency.
Emergency Medical Services (EMS): Community resources and medical personnel that provide emergency care to victims of injury or sudden illness.

Float plan: A written plan with details of a boating trip, left with someone ashore.
Liability: A legal responsibility.
Standard of care: The degree of care expected from a reasonable and careful person under the same or similar circumstances.

INTRODUCTION

Boats can transport people to exciting new environments. People of all ages, levels of experience, and ability enjoy the satisfaction and exhilaration of boating. With good planning and supervision, boating can be safe and fun. This chapter will teach you the importance of small craft trip planning, supervision, and emergency preparation.

SMALL CRAFT TRIP PLANNING

Planning a safe and enjoyable trip includes—

- Selecting a leader.
- Knowing the responsibilities and legal considerations.
- Selecting the locale and route.
- Checking the weather conditions.
- Checking the water conditions.
- Choosing the appropriate clothing.
- Selecting and checking the appropriate equipment.
- Preparing for possible emergencies.

Selecting a Leader

A group leader should be a responsible person with leadership experience, safety training, and good judgment. He or she should have experience in an environment similar to the group's destination. The group leader should be able to guide the group through all phases of the trip, and take charge if a crisis arises. *Do not attempt a trip without competent leadership.*

Responsibilities and Legal Considerations

As a group leader, you are responsible for the safety of trip participants. To help provide for the safety of the participants, consider their limits, skill levels, and experience. Be aware of and responsive to medical conditions or restrictions that participants may have. Ask participants to tell you their abilities, limitations, and other considerations.

Regardless of ability, people share the same need for fun, adventure, and skill development. Simple adaptations can help all people enjoy small craft activities. It is best to meet each individual's needs and focus on the participant's ability, not disability.

Providing for the safety of small craft participants with disabilities is similar to providing for the safety of small craft participants without disabilities. Certain accommodations and adjustments need to be made, depending on the participant's ability, type of craft, and water environment. The prevention of small craft accidents, injuries, and fatalities through proper trip planning, supervision, and emergency preparation is the best way to help provide for everyone's safety.

Being a group leader involves some legal responsibility, or *liability*. Group leaders should have a thorough understanding of the responsibilities and legal implications of supervising a group. This information can help prevent accidents and **negligence** which may result in a **lawsuit**.

Group leaders—both volunteer and paid—are legally accountable for their actions and may be responsible for the actions of group members as well. They need to know the policies and procedures of the facility or organization with which they are associated.

Group leaders may be required to have certain training and certifications. They are expected to provide a *standard of care* that includes accepting responsibility for minimizing risks and responding quickly and appropriately in emergency situations. Specific responsibilities of group leaders are set by an employer, organization, or other governing agency and should be communicated to and understood by the group leader.

Selecting the Locale and Route

The location, duration, and difficulty of the trip should depend on the capabilities of the group, type of craft, and weather conditions. Keep in mind the limits of your ability and the group members' abilities. If the trip is beyond your ability or the abilities of your group members, change the trip plan.

Detailed planning makes trips safer. Guidebooks that include information about possible campsites, known hazards, river classifications, and **portage** trails are a good source of information for small craft trips. Printed reference materials, maps, and navigation charts are often available through local, state, or federal agencies.

Before departing, fill out a *float plan*. This plan should include the following information:

- Names of group members
- Starting point
- Route and checkpoints
- Destination
- Planned return time
- Whom to contact if you do not return as scheduled

A float plan is particularly important if you are traveling in a wilderness area, or if you plan to be gone for an extended period of time. Give the float plan to a responsible person, and ask him or her to contact the local Coast Guard or law enforcement agency if you do not return as scheduled. (See Appendix D for a sample float plan.)

Checking the Weather Conditions

Storms, high winds, and fog are dangerous to boaters. Check the weather forecast in the local newspaper and on local radio or television stations. Consider delaying or postponing your trip if you encounter any of the following signs of bad weather:

- Growing cloud cover and darkening skies
- Sudden changes in wind velocity or direction, or gusty winds

CHAPTER 2   *Trip Planning, Supervision, and Emergency Preparation*

- Lightning
- Thunder
- Increasing waves
- Sudden temperature changes

If a storm approaches while you are on the water—

- Return to shore at the first sound of thunder or flash of lightning, regardless of how far away it seems. Water conducts the electricity of lightning.
- Seek shelter in an enclosed area.
- Stay away from open areas, trees, and tall or metal objects.
- If you are caught in a boat during a storm and unable to return to shore, stay as low as possible in the craft.

Checking the Water Conditions

Good weather does not automatically mean that water conditions are good. The weather may be sunny, clear, and calm—yet a river's water could be dangerously fast and cold because of recent rains or snow melt. The water level of many lakes and rivers is controlled by dams and can change quickly. Water conditions can also be affected by tides,

Lightning

Approximately 100 times each second,[1] a lightning bolt strikes the earth. (Lightning bolts can generate temperatures that are hotter than the surface of the sun—up to 50,000 degrees F.[2]) Each year, lightning strikes in the United States kill about 100 people and injure about 300 more.[3]

The explosive shock wave generated by the lightning bolt causes the noise that we call "thunder." If you can hear thunder, you can be struck by lightning. Whenever you hear thunder, leave the water immediately and seek safe shelter. Stay in a safe place for 15 minutes after you last hear thunder or see lightning.

A safe shelter might be—

- Inside a sturdy building (not an isolated shed or a picnic shelter).
- Inside an all-metal car (not a convertible).

If shelter is unavailable follow these guidelines:

- Get out of the boat and away from the water.
- Find the lowest spot possible, and avoid trees, poles, or other objects that project above the terrain.
- If in a group, spread out and stay away from any metal gear or equipment.

In any case, stay away from water and grounded metal objects that conduct electricity, including fences, pipes, electric appliances, telephones, and metal sheds. If your skin begins to tingle or your hair feels like it's standing on end, assume the "lightning safe position."[4] Squat or crouch as low as possible, with your knees drawn up, both feet together, and hands off the ground.

Do not lie flat on the ground; minimize ground contact.

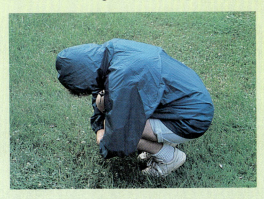

If someone is struck by lightning, give first aid immediately. Most people struck by lightning stop breathing and suffer serious injuries, yet survive. Outdoor activity leaders should be trained in first aid and CPR and be able to give proper care in emergencies.

To help avoid lightning strikes, listen to National Oceanic and Atmospheric Administration (NOAA) weather radio, commercial radio, or television weather reports before your outing. Be alert for these warnings:

- A severe thunderstorm *watch* tells you when and where thunderstorms are most likely to occur.
- A severe thunderstorm *warning* tells you that severe weather has already been reported by spotters or indicated by radar.

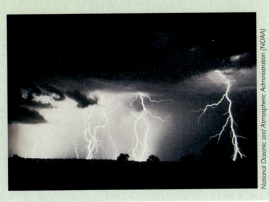

---

[1] L. Michael Trapasso and Greg Owens, *Eye to the Sky: Understanding the Danger of Thunderstorms and Lightning* (Parks & Recreation), August 1996, Vol. 31, No. 8, pp. 62-67.

[2] *Thunderstorms and Lightning, the Underrated Killers!* (NOAA and the American Red Cross), January 1994.

[3] Trapasso and Owens, *Eye to the Sky: Understanding the Danger of Thunderstorms and Lightning*.

[4] Ibid.

currents, and other hazards. Proper planning includes finding out about these conditions and potential hazards ahead of time.

Choosing the Appropriate Equipment

Some of the factors to consider when choosing equipment include the duration of the trip, type of water, weather conditions, remoteness of location, and potential portages. Take equipment that is in good shape, and practice using the equipment before the trip. Consider bringing the following:

Group items

- Matches in a waterproof container
- Flashlight with extra bulbs and batteries
- Tent or other shelter
- Food and cooking gear
- Water purification tablets or filter
- Maps, charts, and compass
- Portable radio for weather reports
- Boat repair kit
- Tools, such as pliers and screwdrivers
- Duct tape

Personal items

- Toiletry kit
- Head and eye gear, such as a hat, helmet, and sunglasses
- Extra clothes in waterproof bags
- Rain gear
- Dry suit or wet suit
- Ground cloth
- Sleeping bag
- Sleeping pad
- Waterproof packs
- Footwear
- Drinking water
- Toilet paper
- Sunscreen and insect repellent

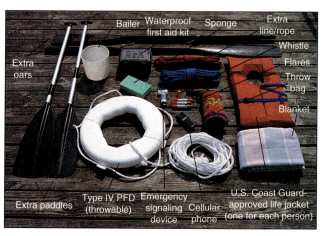

Figure 2-1

Safety Equipment

Regardless of the type of boat, make sure that you have the basic safety equipment on board. The exact equipment required depends on federal, regional, and state laws; the type of small craft; and the location and duration of your trip. A basic list includes the following (Fig. 2-1):

- A U.S. Coast Guard-approved life jacket for each person on board
- A Type IV (throwable) PFD
- A throw bag
- Extra line/rope
- Extra paddles/oars
- Bailers and sponges
- A first aid kit in a waterproof container
- Blankets
- A means of communication, such as a cellular phone or two-way radio
- A sound device, such as an air horn or whistle
- A visual distress signal, such as a flare, strobe light, signal mirror, chemical light stick, or colored dye marker

Checking the Craft and Equipment

Before starting your trip, check your boat and equipment to make sure they are in good working order.

- Test new and unfamiliar equipment.
- Make certain that the craft is in good repair. On a multiday trip, check the craft at the beginning of each day.
- Make sure that the paddles or oars are strong and properly sized.
- Install safety lines that you can hold onto in case your craft capsizes. These lines may also aid in craft recovery.
- Make sure all lines and equipment are properly secured to avoid entanglement while operating your craft.
- Make sure the craft is not overloaded.
- Make sure you have appropriate repair materials and equipment.

Helmets and Paddling

In certain types of water you should wear a helmet specially designed for paddling. Kayakers paddling a decked craft generally wear helmets to protect their heads when they roll. Canoers using **thigh straps**, paddling a decked craft, or canoeing difficult rapids often wear helmets as well. It is important to take into account the type of water, craft, activity, and ability of participants when making a decision about helmet use. If you are instructing or leading paddling activities for an organization, check with the organization for specific guidelines regarding helmet use.

If you and your group are wearing helmets, make sure they are designed for paddling, and that they are properly sized and fitted.

CHAPTER 2   *Trip Planning, Supervision, and Emergency Preparation*

Choosing the Appropriate Clothing

Choose clothing that preserves body heat even when wet. Consider a layer of insulating clothing (wool, **polypropylene, capalene**) under a jacket and pants made of a light, waterproof fabric like a paddle suit. This provides insulation for warmth, helps shed water, and reduces heat loss from wind and evaporation.

Another option is a wet suit or dry suit. Many frequent boaters invest in some wet suit components like a vest, shorts, and booties.

Wear shoes to keep you from slipping, and to protect your feet from cuts and other injuries. Avoid wearing heavy or bulky footwear such as boots. Wear a hat to protect your face from the sun and keep your head warm.

SMALL CRAFT SUPERVISION

There are a number of elements to supervising small craft participants safely and effectively. These include effective communication, safe leader-to-participant ratios, and proper supervisor location.

Communication

Good communication is necessary for boating safety, regardless of whether you're in a canoe, kayak, sailboat, or rowboat. Before starting a small craft outing, communicate the following to participants:

- Each participant's responsibilities
- Safety rules for participants
- Where and how far craft may travel
- Emergency signals to be used, such as whistle blows or hand signals
- Distance between craft

Effective communication is essential for everyone's safety on the water. Regardless of the type of craft, communicate the following information to your passengers and to other craft:

- Announce any sudden changes in direction.
- Warn fellow boaters of objects or other craft that need to be avoided.
- Warn passengers of any wake, waves, or rapids that are coming up.
- Advise others on board if you need to move or change positions.
- Advise other craft in your group if they are too far away, too far ahead, or falling behind.

Leader-to-Participant Ratios

Many camps, agencies, and outfitters establish leader-to-participant ratios for small craft activities. These ratios are set to provide adequate supervision and participant safety.

Check with your state or local boating administrator for leader-to-participant ratios. If no ratios are established, consider the following factors in determining leader-to-participant ratios for small craft activities:

- Number of craft being supervised
- Number of participants being supervised
- Age and ability of participants
- Type of craft being supervised
- Type of water and weather conditions
- Type, duration, and location of the activity

Leader Location

Proper location of small craft leaders will help provide effective supervision. The same factors that determine adequate leader-to-participant ratios need to be considered when determining leader location; the number of craft and participants being supervised; the age and ability of participants; the type of craft; water and weather conditions; and the type, duration, and location of the activity. There are several options:

- The leader may be in the **lead craft**—the front or first craft. The lead craft should have someone in it who has previously navigated the waters and is familiar with the area.
- The leader may be in the **sweep craft**—the craft that brings up the rear to ensure that no one is left behind.
- The leader may be in the **safety boat**, also known as the chase boat. From a safety boat, a number of small craft can be observed, and any craft that stray too far can be retrieved.
- The leader may elect to move among the various craft to ensure all is well and to offer any instructions or answer questions.

EMERGENCY PREPARATION

Being prepared for an emergency means being ready *before* it happens. Although you cannot foresee every water-related emergency, following the water safety guidelines in the Introduction (see page 2) should help prevent emergencies from occurring. If an emergency *does* occur, being prepared may help lower the risk of serious injury or death.

To be prepared for an emergency, you must first understand the aquatic environment you will be in. Always—

- Be aware of the conditions and potential hazards of the water environment whether it is a lake, river, ocean, or other body of water. Know its unique conditions, as well as hazards common in your geographical area, such as storms, currents, and underwater obstructions.
- Understand the various recreational activities that are common in the water environment. Consider the age and ability of participants in those activities.

SMALL CRAFT SAFETY

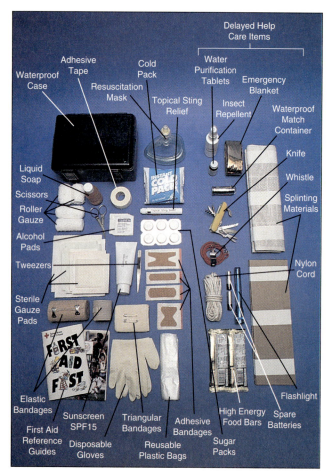

Figure 2-2

- Learn what kind of accidents and injuries have occurred in the past in the water environment. This knowledge will help you prevent further injuries, and be prepared for similar aquatic emergencies.
- Have the appropriate safety equipment (see page 14) and first aid supplies for the water environment (Fig. 2-2).

Emergency Action Plan

When responding to an emergency, you should have a plan to direct your actions. This is called an *emergency action plan (EAP)*. It includes appropriate steps to follow when an emergency occurs. An EAP should be—

- Simple.
- Easy to remember.
- In writing and clearly understood by everyone in the group.

The plan should be discussed and practiced regularly so that everyone knows what to do. For example, if a craft car-rying several people capsizes and everyone falls into the water, will everyone know what to do? Will the group leader know what to do if one of the people is not found immediately? Knowing exactly what to do in an emergency can help prevent serious injury and possibly save lives.

Developing an Emergency Action Plan

An EAP should be developed for any emergency that could occur in a small craft activity. An EAP includes these general features:

- How the person who recognizes the emergency is to signal others
- The steps each person in the group should take in an emergency
- The location of rescue and safety equipment
- Actions to minimize the emergency and safely rescue any victims
- How to call for medical assistance when needed
- Follow-up procedures after an emergency

Before writing your EAP, talk with fellow staff members, volunteer leaders, and participants. If you belong to an agency or organization, check its safety guidelines or consult with the safety officer.

Most emergency action plans include steps for managing specific types of emergencies. For example, an incident involving multiple victims may require coordinating the efforts of different group members.

Contents of an Emergency Action Plan

An emergency action plan should include the following content areas as appropriate:

▶ Layout of facility/environment
  - **Emergency Medical Services (EMS)** access and entry/exit routes
  - Location of rescue and first aid equipment
  - Location of telephones, with emergency telephone numbers posted
  - Exits and evacuation routes

▶ Equipment available
  - Rescue equipment
  - First aid supplies
  - Emergency equipment

▶ Support personnel
  - Internal
    + Staff members
    + Volunteer leaders
    + Participants
  - External
    + EMS personnel (police officers and fire fighters)
    + Search and rescue team and local Coast Guard
    + Hospitals

▶ Staff Responsibilities
  - Assign each person or staff member a duty—

CHAPTER 2   *Trip Planning, Supervision, and Emergency Preparation*   17

When Help Is Delayed

When emergency medical care is delayed 30 minutes or more it is called a delayed-help situation. This delay exists because there may be no easy way—

- To call for help.
- For emergency personnel to reach the victim.
- To transport the victim to medical care.

When planning a trip in a delayed-help environment, several major considerations will help you determine special safety needs. These include—

- How many people in the group know first aid for delayed-help environments and CPR?
- How many people are trained in water safety?
- What is the maximum anticipated delay in obtaining medical help?
- What is the total duration of the trip or activity?
- What is the level of risk associated with the activity and environment?
- Do any group members have preexisting medical or physical conditions?
- What special equipment and supplies are needed?
- How many people are in the group?

If an emergency occurs in the wilderness, you may need to improvise or modify the care you provide, depending on the environment and the circumstances. You will need to spend more time caring for the victim and monitoring his or her condition while waiting for help.

You need to consider how you are going to get help. Should you—

- Stay where you are and call, radio, or signal for help?
- Send someone to get help or leave the victim alone to go get help?
- Transport the victim to get help?

+ Provide care.
+ Warn other craft of emergency.
+ Meet EMS personnel.
+ Interview witnesses.

▶ Communication
- Means available to obtain medical help or access to call 9-1-1
- The local emergency number, and who will make the call
- Chain of command
- Person to contact family/guardian
- Person to deal with media

▶ Follow-up
- This includes items such as EAP evaluation and documentation. See the following section, "After an Emergency," for a detailed description of follow-up items.

After an Emergency

When the emergency is over you may need to complete follow-up procedures. For example, you may be responsible for—

- Confirming that witnesses have been interviewed and their observations documented.
- Reporting the incident to the appropriate individual (this may be your supervisor) or authorities.
- Contacting a victim's family/guardian.
- Dealing with the media.
- Inspecting equipment and supplies used in the emergency. Make sure that all equipment used is back in place and in good working condition. Replace any used supplies.
- Filling out any report forms and transmitting the reports appropriately.
- Conducting a debriefing or arranging a critical incident stress debriefing (see page 19).
- Assessing what happened and evaluating the actions taken. You should—
  – Review the event as a group.
  – Consider what worked well and what could have worked better.
  – Change the EAP to correct any weak areas.
  – Practice the new plan as soon as possible.

Reports

All injuries and incidents should be documented and reported appropriately.

These reports may be used for insurance purposes and in a court of law. Some agencies or organizations may already have a form for this purpose. If not, one can be developed from the examples on page 18.

INSTRUCTIONS FOR EMERGENCY TELEPHONE CALLS

Emergency telephone numbers
(dial _____ for outside line)
EMS: _____
Fire: _____
Police: _____
Poison Control Center: _____
Number of this telephone: _____

Other Important Telephone Numbers
Facility manager: _____
Facility maintenance: _____
Power company: _____
Gas company: _____
Weather bureau: _____
Name and address of medical facility with 24-hour emergency cardiac care: _____
_____

Information for Emergency Call
(Be prepared to give this information to the EMS dispatcher)
1. Location: _____
   Street address _____
   City or town _____
   Directions (cross streets, roads, landmarks, etc.): _____
   _____
2. Telephone number from which the call is being made
   _____
3. Caller's name _____
4. What happened _____
5. How many people are injured _____
6. Condition of injured person(s) _____
7. Help (care) being provided _____

Note: Do not hang up first. Let the EMS dispatcher hang up first.

Note: In cities with Enhanced 9-1-1 (9-1-1E) systems, it is still important to know the information above for communication to the dispatcher. In many buildings, the telephone system may connect through a switchboard that will show only the corporate address rather than the specific facility from which you are calling. With cellular telephones, 9-1-1E is not functional in identifying a fixed location on the dispatcher's screen. Sharing this information is the only way to provide it.

(Sample form—post by telephone)

SAMPLE INCIDENT REPORT FORM

Date of report: _____ Date of incident: _____
Time of incident: _____

Facility Information
Facility: _____ Phone #: _____
Address: _____ City _____
State _____ Zip _____

Personal Data - Injured Party
Name: _____ Age: ____ Gender: _____
Address: _____ City _____
State _____ Zip _____
Phone number(s): home: _____
                 work: _____
Family contact (name and phone #): _____

Incident Data
Location of incident: _____
Description of incident: _____
Was an injury sustained: Yes ____ No ____
If yes, describe the type of injury sustained: _____
Witnesses _____
  1. Name: _____ Phone #: _____
     Address: _____ City _____
     State _____ Zip _____
  2. Name: _____ Phone #: _____
     Address: _____ City _____
     State _____ Zip _____

Care Provided
Did victim refuse medical attention by staff?
                                Yes ____ No ____
Was care provided by facility staff? Yes ____ No ____
Name of the person who provided care: _____
Describe in detail care provided: _____
_____
Were universal precautions taken: Yes ____ No ____
Was EMS called? _____
If yes, by whom? _____ Time EMS called: _____
                                Time EMS arrived: _____
Was the victim transported to an emergency facility? ____
If yes, where? _____
If no, person returned to activity? Yes ____ No ____
If no, what was the referral action taken: _____

Victim's signature (Parent's/Guardian's if victim is a minor):
_____ Date: _____

Facility Data
Number of staff on duty at time of incident: _____
Weather conditions at time of incident: _____
Conditions at time of incident: _____
Name(s) of staff involved in incident: _____

Report Prepared By:
Name (please print): _____
Position: _____
Signature: _____

CHAPTER 2 *Trip Planning, Supervision, and Emergency Preparation* 19

Critical Incident Stress

An emergency involving a serious injury or death is a critical incident. The acute stress it causes an individual can overcome his or her ability to cope. This acute stress is called *critical incident stress.*

Some effects of critical incident stress may appear right away and others may appear after days, weeks, or even months have passed. People suffering from critical incident stress may not be able to perform their jobs well. If not managed properly, this acute stress may lead to a serious condition called post-traumatic stress disorder.

Signs of critical incident stress include the following:

- Confusion
- Lowered attention span; restlessness
- Denial
- Guilt or depression
- Anger
- Anxiety
- Changes in interactions with others
- Increased or decreased eating (weight gain or weight loss)
- Uncharacteristic, excessive humor or silence
- Unusual behavior
- Sleeplessness
- Nightmares

Critical incident stress requires professional help to prevent post-traumatic stress disorder. An individual can reduce stress by—

- Practicing relaxation techniques.
- Eating a balanced diet.
- Avoiding caffeine, alcohol, and drugs.
- Getting enough rest.
- Participating in some type of physical exercise or activity.

Critical Incident Stress Debriefing

A process called critical incident stress debriefing (CISD) brings together a group of people experiencing critical incident stress with some of their peers, such as other staff members, and a trained mental health professional. This process helps those with critical incident stress share and understand their feelings while learning to cope.

Emergency service agencies usually have CISD teams trained to respond and give critical incident stress debriefings. Emergency action plans should include information on obtaining help for managing critical incident stress.

For more information on CISD and stress management, contact: Critical Incident Stress Foundation, 10176 Baltimore National Pike, Suite 201, Ellicott City, Maryland 21042-3652, (410) 750-9600, or a local mental health professional.

SUMMARY

A group leader for a boating trip has many responsibilities, including the safety of trip participants. When planning a trip, both the leader and participants must make informed decisions. It is important to know the local weather patterns and the aquatic environment. Make sure you have the proper equipment—including first aid and rescue equipment—and know how to use it. Know how to prepare and maintain the water craft. Above all, write an emergency action plan (EAP) and practice it regularly so that everyone knows their role in an emergency.

LEARNING ACTIVITIES

TRUE OR FALSE

Circle the correct answer.

1. A group leader cannot be held responsible for the actions of group members.   True or False?

2. The location, duration, and difficulty of the trip should primarily depend on the skill and experience of the group members.   True or False?

3. If the weather is fair, you can assume that water conditions are favorable.   True or False?

4. An emergency action plan should be understood by everyone in the group.   True or False?

5. An emergency action plan should be detailed and cover any emergency that could occur in planned small craft activities.   True or False?

MULTIPLE CHOICE

Circle the letter of the best answer or answers.

1. Necessary skills of a group leader include—
   a. Leadership experience and safety training.
   b. Weather forecasting.
   c. The ability to take charge in a crisis.
   d. Experience in an environment similar to the group's destination.
   e. a, c, and d.

2. A good float plan includes—
   a. Names of the group members.
   b. Starting point, checkpoints, and destination.
   c. Approximate time of arrival at destination.
   d. Whom to contact if you do not return as scheduled.
   e. All of the above.

3. Which of the following items is NOT a guideline to follow before an aquatic outing?
   a. Check manufacturer's warranty.
   b. Test new and unfamiliar equipment.
   c. Secure all lines and equipment to avoid entanglements.
   d. Make sure the craft is not overloaded.
   e. Make sure appropriate repair materials are on board.

4. An emergency action plan should include the following:
   a. How to signal members of the group that an emergency has occurred
   b. The location of rescue equipment
   c. Reporting an incident to the media
   d. a and b

5. The primary way incident reports may help prevent similar incidents in the future is by—
   a. Serving as a legal document, which may be used in court.
   b. Fulfilling a requirement of federal, state, and/or local government.
   c. Providing a record that can be reviewed to make an activity or outing safer.
   d. Identifying who was at fault.
   e. Punishing those found at fault.

FILL IN

Fill in the correct answers.

1. List at least four signs of possible bad weather:
   _____
   _____
   _____
   _____

2. Prior to embarking on a boating excursion, you should fill out a _____ and give it to a responsible person.

3. Basic boating safety equipment includes (list four or more): _____
   _____
   _____
   _____
   _____

CHAPTER 2 *Trip Planning, Supervision, and Emergency Preparation*

SCENARIO

1. You have been asked to make sure the annual employee canoe trip down a local river is a safe event.

   a. List four points of emergency preparation:
      1. _____
      2. _____
      3. _____
      4. _____

   b. Basic safety equipment includes, a first aid kit, means of communication, and visual distress signal. Other safety equipment the group should carry includes (list at least three)—
      _____
      _____
      _____

   c. What are some important steps you need to take to plan for a safe and enjoyable trip? (list at least three)—
      _____
      _____
      _____

   d. What information about the participants should you consider when planning a trip? (list at least three)—
      _____
      _____
      _____

See answers to learning activities on pages 82–83.

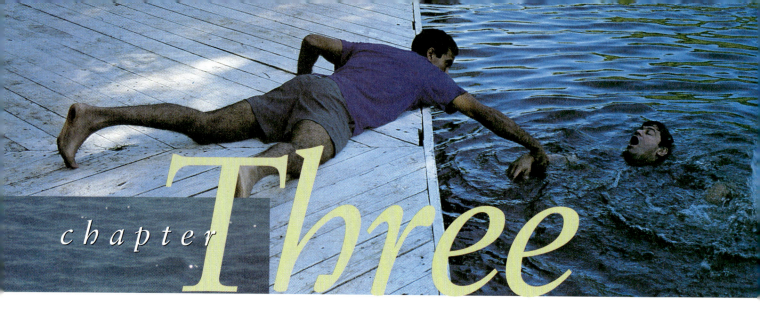

chapter Three

Basic Water Rescue

OBJECTIVES

After reading this chapter you should be able to—
1. Describe survival floating in warm water.
2. Describe how to trap air in your clothing for buoyancy.
3. Describe what you can do to prevent or delay hypothermia.
4. Describe what to do if you fall into water without a life jacket.
5. Recognize the characteristics of distressed swimmers and active and passive drowning victims.
6. Identify at least three situations in which a head, neck, or back injury should be suspected.
7. Identify at least five signals of a head, neck, or back injury.
8. Describe the five guidelines for caring for a head, neck, or back injury.
9. Describe how to assist someone having a seizure in the water.
10. Explain the importance of emergency care after a victim is out of the water.
11. Define the key terms for this chapter.

After reading this chapter and completing the appropriate course activities, you should be able to—
1. Demonstrate the HELP and huddle positions.
2. Demonstrate two reaching assists.
3. Demonstrate throwing assists using two different pieces of equipment.
4. Demonstrate the wading assist, the walking assist, and the beach drag.
5. Demonstrate two ways to stabilize a victim's head, neck, and back in the water.

KEY TERMS

Active drowning victim: A person exhibiting universal behavior that includes struggling at the surface for 20 to 60 seconds before submerging.
Distressed swimmer: A person capable of staying afloat but likely to need assistance to get to safety.
Emergency Medical Services (EMS) personnel: Trained and equipped community-based personnel dispatched through an emergency number, usually 9-1-1, to provide medical care to victims of injury or sudden illness.
Hypothermia: A life-threatening condition in which the body is unable to maintain warmth and the entire body cools.
Passive drowning victim: An unconscious victim facedown, submerged, or near the surface of the water.

INTRODUCTION

It is not uncommon for boaters to end up in the water unexpectedly. In this chapter you will learn how to rescue yourself and others from the water in different situations. You will also learn what to do when special situations occur, such as head, neck, and back injuries, or **seizures**.

SELF-RESCUE

Self-rescue skills are important for any person who may find himself or herself in the water unexpectedly and may be unable to reach help immediately. If you find yourself in water and are wearing a life jacket, you can stay safe on the surface until you reach safety or are rescued by others. If you are in the water without a life jacket and you cannot reach safety, do not panic. You can use different methods to stay afloat while awaiting rescue or making your way to safety.

If you can swim, use a stroke that keeps your arms in the water, such as the breaststroke, sidestroke, or elementary backstroke. Swim in a way that is most comfortable for you. Perfect strokes are not necessary to keep from sinking. Tread water or float while you try to signal for help, and wait to be rescued.

The next sections describe survival floating and two ways to trap air in your clothing for buoyancy in case you find yourself in the water without a life jacket. Practice these so that you are prepared for an emergency.

Survival Floating

Survival floating is floating facedown in *warm water*. Use this method if you cannot reach safety and need to wait for help, or need to rest while making your way to safety.

When facedown in the water, your body tends to swing down to a nearly vertical position, with your head at or just below the surface. Survival floating is based on this natural position. It helps someone in warm water save energy while waiting to be rescued. By making slow and easy movements with your arms and legs, you can stay afloat in this position for a long period of time.

1. Hold your breath and put your face in the water. Allow your arms and legs to hang freely. Rest in this position for a few seconds (Fig. 3-1, A).
2. To take a breath, slowly lift your arms to about shoulder height and move your arms forward. Separate your legs, moving one leg forward and one leg back.
3. Gently press down with your arms and at the same time bring your legs together. This movement lifts your mouth above water, allowing you to take another breath (Fig. 3-1, B).
4. Return to the resting position. Repeat these movements to take the next breath.

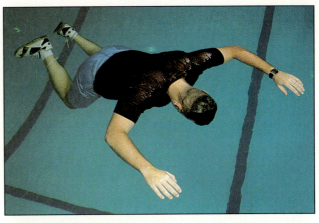
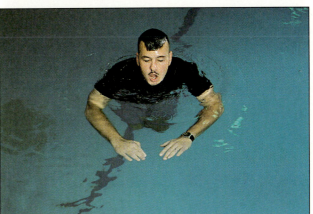

Figure 3-1, A and B

Self-Rescue When Clothed

Water emergencies can happen even when you do not intend to go in the water. If you find yourself in the water unexpectedly, leave your clothes on. Most clothing can help you float. If you can float wearing your shoes, leave them on. If they are too heavy, remove them.

If you are wearing a long-sleeved shirt or jacket, try to trap air in the shoulders to help keep you afloat. Use either of the following methods to get air into your shirt or jacket for flotation:

Method 1
Use this method to inflate your shirt or jacket by blowing air into it.

1. While treading water, tuck your shirt or jacket in, or tie the shirttail ends together.
2. Unbutton the collar button, take a deep breath, bend your head forward into the water, pull the shirt or jacket up to your face, and blow into the shirt (Fig. 3-2, A).
3. Keep the front of the shirt or jacket underwater and hold the collar closed. The air will rise and form a bubble in the shoulders of the shirt or jacket (Fig. 3-2, B).
4. Repeat the steps to reinflate the shirt or jacket, if necessary.

Small Craft Safety

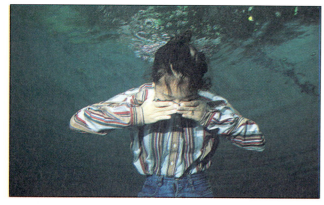
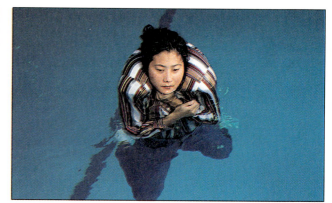

Figure 3-2, A and B

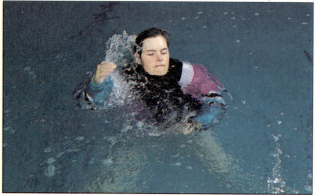

Figure 3-3, A and B

Method 2

Use this method to inflate your shirt or jacket by splashing air into it.

1. While treading water, fasten the top buttons of the shirt or zip the jacket up to the neck.
2. Hold the front bottom of the shirt or jacket out with one hand, keeping it just under the surface of the water. Lean back slightly.
3. From above the surface, strike the water with your free hand (palm down) and drive it down to a point below the shirttail or jacket. The air carried down from the surface will bubble into the shirt or jacket (Fig. 3-3, A).
4. Keep the front of the shirt or jacket underwater and hold the collar and shirttail closed. The air will rise and form a bubble in the shoulders of the shirt or jacket (Fig. 3-3, B).
5. Repeat the steps to reinflate the shirt or jacket, if necessary.

You may also use your pants to help keep you afloat if you are in *warm water*.

1. Take a deep breath, lean forward into the water, reach down, and remove your shoes.
2. While treading water, loosen the waistband and/or belt of your pants.
3. Again, take a deep breath, lean forward, reach down, and take off your pants one leg at a time. Bring your face to the surface and take a breath whenever you need one. Do not hurry (Fig. 3-4, A).
4. Once the pants are off, tie both legs together at the cuff, or tie a knot in each leg as close as you can to the bottom of the leg (Fig. 3-4, B). Then zip or button the pants to the waist.
5. Hold the back of the waistband underwater with one hand, and with the pants on the surface, splash air into the open waistband with your free hand. Splash the air in by striking down with the palm of your hand and following through to below the waistband held open below the surface (Fig. 3-4, C).
6. You can also inflate your pants by submerging and blowing air into them through the open waistband underwater (Fig. 3-5).
7. When the pants are inflated, gather the waistband together either in your hands, or by tightening the belt. Slip your head between the pant legs where they are tied together. If the pant legs are tied separately, reach one arm over and between the two pant legs for support (Fig. 3-6, A, B).
8. Repeat the steps to reinflate the pants, if necessary.

CHAPTER 3   Basic Water Rescue   25

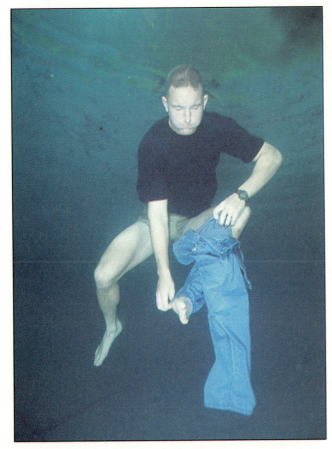
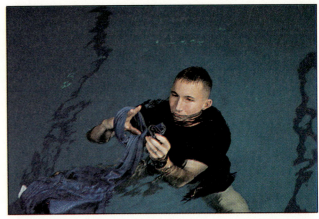
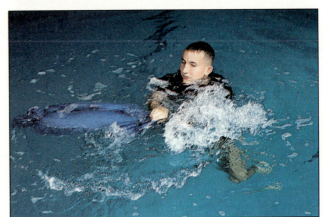

Figure 3-4, A, B and C

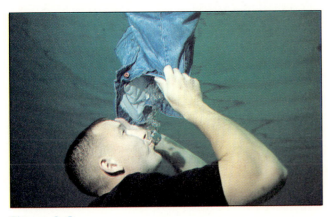

Figure 3-5

Self-Rescue When Wearing a Life Jacket

If you fall into deep water wearing a life jacket—

1. Keep your face and head above the surface. If you are near a capsized boat or large debris, such as logs or boards, climb as far out of the water as you can onto the boat or debris. Get as much of your body out of the water as possible.

2. Keep all your clothes on, especially your hat. Even wet clothes help maintain your body heat.

    In cold water, you must decide between trying to reach safety or floating while waiting for help. Remember that you cannot swim as far in cold water as in warm water. If you can reach safety with a few strokes, do so. If not, float and wait to be rescued. If you swim, use strokes that will keep your arms underwater, such as the breaststroke or sidestroke. Keeping your arms underwater uses less energy.

HELP Position

HELP stands for Heat Escape Lessening Posture. This position is used by one person wearing a life jacket to conserve body heat in cold water while awaiting rescue.

1. Draw your knees up to your chest.
2. Keep your face forward and out of the water.
3. Hold your upper arms at your sides, and hold your lower arms against or across your chest (Fig. 3-7).

Do not use the HELP position in moving water.

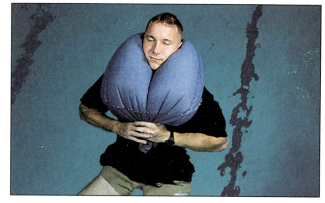
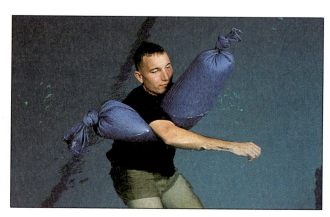

Figure 3-6, A and B

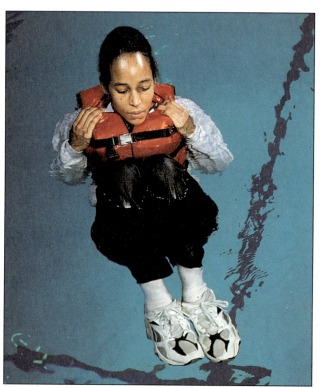

Figure 3-7

Figure 3-8

Huddle Position

The **huddle position** is for two or more people wearing life jackets to conserve body heat in *cold water* while awaiting rescue.

- With two people, put your arms around each other so that your chests are together.
- With three or more people, put your arms over each other's shoulders so that the sides of your chests are together (Fig. 3-8). Place children or elderly persons in the middle of the huddle.

Do not use the huddle position in fast-moving water.

RESCUING OTHERS

You need to know how to rescue others from the water in addition to yourself. This starts with recognizing when an emergency is happening.

Recognizing Aquatic Emergencies

An emergency can happen to anyone in, on, or around the water. Emergencies can occur regardless of how experienced the boater is or how good of a swimmer the person is. A boater may have trouble in the water because of a sudden unexpected fall, capsize, or collision.

Recognizing that a person is having trouble in the water may help save his or her life. People slip underwater quickly without calling for help. Therefore, you need to recognize that a person may be in trouble before it is

CHAPTER 3   Basic Water Rescue   27

too late. Table 3-1 summarizes how to recognize *distressed swimmers* and *active* and *passive drowning victims*.

Rescue Guidelines

Knowing how to help others in the water is important. Always act safely to reduce the risk of becoming a victim yourself. To stay safe when helping someone in trouble, do not enter the water.

If you must assist someone who is having trouble in the water, you must have appropriate equipment for your own safety and the victim's. For example, wear a life jacket when helping someone in open water. If the appropriate safety equipment is not available and there is a chance that you cannot safely help a person in trouble, call for immediate assistance.

Note: Swimming into deep water to bring a victim to shore requires special training (for example, lifeguard training) and equipment. Do not swim out to a victim without the proper training and equipment. You can put yourself in danger and risk two lives rather than saving one.

Reaching Assist with Equipment

If a victim is close enough, without going into the water yourself, use a **reaching assist** to help him or her out of the water. Use any object to extend your reach, such as a pole,

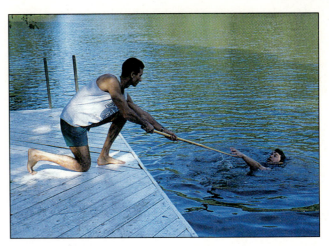

Figure 3-9

a **shepherd's crook**, an oar, a paddle, a tree branch, a shirt, a belt, or a towel. Follow these steps to keep yourself safe:

1. Brace yourself in the craft, on the pier surface, or shoreline.
2. Extend the object to the victim (Fig. 3-9).
3. When the victim grasps the object, slowly and carefully pull him or her to safety. Keep your body low, and lean back to avoid being pulled into the water.

TABLE 3-1

BEHAVIORS	SWIMMER	DISTRESSED SWIMMER	ACTIVE DROWNING VICTIM	PASSIVE DROWNING VICTIM
Breathing	Rhythmic breathing	Can continue breathing and call for help	Struggles to breathe; cannot call out for help	Not breathing
Arm and Leg Action	Relatively coordinated movement	Floating, sculling, or treading water; can wave for help	Arms to sides alternately moving up and pressing down; no supporting kick	None
Body Position	Horizontal	Horizontal, vertical, or diagonal, depending on means of support	Vertical	Facedown, submerged
Locomotion	Recognizable	Little or no forward progress; less and less able to support self	None; has only 20-60 seconds before submerging	None

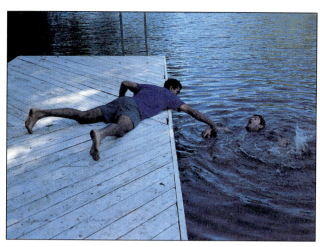

Figure 3-10

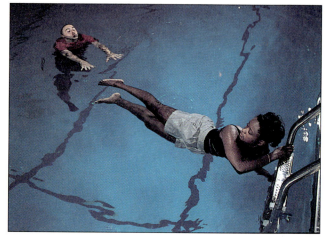

Figure 3-11

Reaching Assist without Equipment

If there is no equipment available to perform a reaching assist, you can—

1. Brace yourself in the craft, on the pier surface, or shoreline.
2. Reach with your arm and grasp the victim (Fig. 3-10).
3. Pull the victim to safety.

If you are already in the water, you can—

1. Hold onto a ladder, pier, piling, or another secure object with one hand.
2. Extend your free hand or one of your legs to the victim (Fig. 3-11). Do not let go of the secure object or swim out into the water.
3. Pull the victim to safety.

Throwing Assist

Use a **throwing assist** to rescue someone from a shoreline or pier who is beyond your reach. Throw the victim a buoyant object tied to a line. He or she can grasp the object and be pulled to safety. Throwing equipment includes U.S. Coast Guard Type IV devices (such as ring buoys and/or buoyant cushions), heaving lines, throw bags, rescue tubes, or any floating object at hand—such as a picnic jug, or extra life jacket. Throwing equipment should be carried on small craft and kept at waterfront areas.

A **throw bag** is a small rescue device often used in small craft. It is a nylon bag with a foam disk and coiled line inside. The disk gives the bag its shape and keeps it from sinking, but it does not provide flotation for someone in the water.

You can make your own **heaving jug** (Fig. 3-12) to keep in your boat and throw to someone having trouble in the water. Put a half-inch of water in a gallon plastic jug, seal it, and attach 50 to 75 feet of floating line to the handle. Hold the handle and throw it with a swinging motion. Release the jug at eye level. The weight of the water in the jug helps carry it to the person in the water (Fig. 3-13).

A heaving line should be made of floating line that is white, yellow, or another easy-to-see color. Tie an object to

Figure 3-12

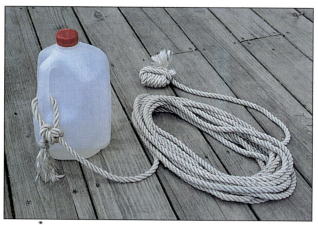

Figure 3-13

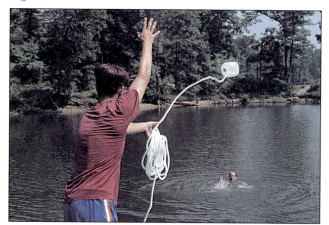

CHAPTER 3   Basic Water Rescue

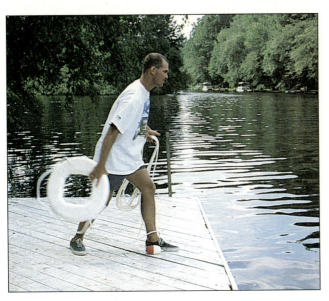

Figure 3-14

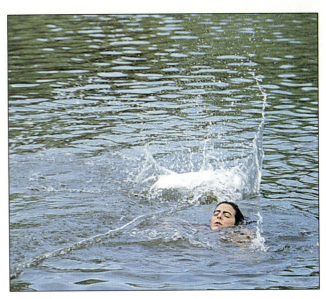

Figure 3-15

Figure 3-16

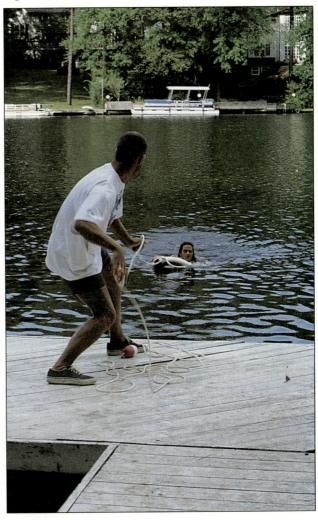

the end of the floating line that has some weight but floats. With about half of the coiled line free to run out from one hand, use the other hand to swing the weighted float in an underhand toss to the person in the water.

A ring buoy is made of cork, **kapok**, cellular foam, or some other buoyant material. It weighs from 3 to 7 pounds. The ring buoy should be attached to a lightweight towline with a large knot at the end to prevent it from slipping out from under your foot when you throw it. Throw the ring buoy underhand.

To perform a throwing assist—

1. Get into a stride position: the leg opposite your throwing arm is forward. This helps to keep your balance when you throw the object (Fig. 3-14).
2. Step on the end of the line with your forward foot.
3. Shout to get the victim's attention. Make eye contact and say that you are going to throw the object now. Tell the victim to grab it.
4. Bend your knees and throw the object to the victim. Try to throw the object upwind and/or up current, just over the victim's head, so the line drops within reach (Fig. 3-15).
5. When the victim has grasped the object or the line, slowly pull him or her to safety (Fig. 3-16). Lean away from the water as you pull.
6. If the object does not reach the victim, quickly pull the line back in and throw it again. Try to keep the line from tangling, but do not waste time trying to recoil it. If the object is a throw bag, partially fill the bag with some water and throw it again.

If the throwing assist does not work, and the water is shallow and safe for wading, try a wading assist with equipment.

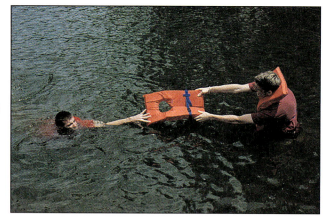
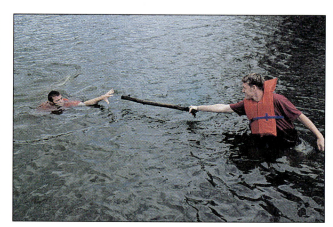

Figure 3-17, A and B

Wading Assist with Equipment

If a current or soft bottom makes wading dangerous, do not go in the water. If the water is safe and shallow enough (not over your chest), you can wade in to reach to the victim. If possible, wear a life jacket. Take something to reach to the victim, such as a—

- Rescue tube.
- Ring buoy.
- Buoyant cushion.
- Kickboard.
- Life jacket.
- Tree branch.
- Pole.
- Air mattress.
- Plastic cooler.
- Picnic jug.
- Paddle.

To perform a wading assist—

1. Take a floating object to extend to the victim.
2. Wade into the water and extend the object to the victim (Fig. 3-17, A, B).
3. When the victim grasps the object, tell him or her to hold on to the object tightly for support, and pull him or her to safety.
4. Keep the object between you and the victim to help prevent him or her from clutching at you in a panic.

Removal from the Water

Sometimes a victim is unconscious or too exhausted to climb or get out of the water. Your decision whether to remove the victim from the water depends on the victim's condition, the length of time before you expect help to arrive, the size of the victim, and the availability of others to help you.

Beach Drag

Use the **beach drag** in shallow water on a sloping shore or beach. This method works well with a heavy or unconscious victim. *Do not use the beach drag if you suspect the victim has a head, neck, or back injury.*

1. Stand behind the victim and grasp him or her under the armpits. Support the head with your forearms.
2. Walk backward slowly and drag the victim onto the shore (Fig. 3-18).
3. Pull the victim completely from the water if you can, or at least get the victim's head and shoulders out of the water.

If someone else is available to help, drag the victim out together as shown in Figure 3-19.

Walking Assist

A victim who is in shallow water and can stand may be able to walk with your help. To use the **walking assist**—

1. Put one of the victim's arms around your neck and over your shoulder.
2. Hold the wrist of the arm that is over your shoulder, and wrap your free arm around the victim's back or waist.
3. Hold the victim firmly, and help him or her walk out of the water (Fig. 3-20).

Figure 3-18

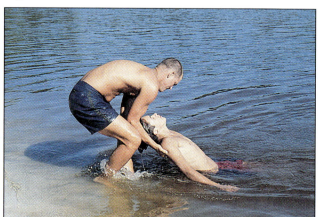

CHAPTER 3   Basic Water Rescue   31

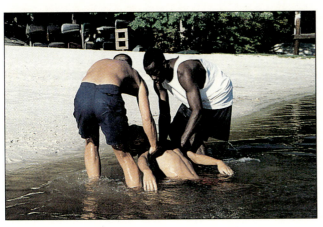

Figure 3-19

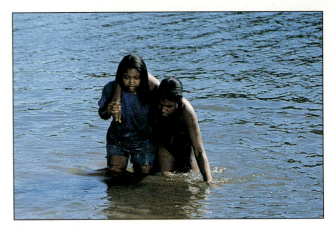

Figure 3-20

EMERGENCY CARE

Head, Neck, and Back Injury

An injury can happen anywhere on the head, neck, or back. Neck injuries most commonly occur when a person dives into shallow water and hits the bottom or strikes an object head-first.

Always suspect a head, neck, or back injury in the following situations:

- Any fall from a height greater than the person's height
- Any person found unconscious for an unknown reason
- Any serious head injury
- Any injury from using a diving board or water slide, or from diving from a height, such as a bank or a cliff
- Diving into shallow water

Always be alert to these signals of head, neck, or back injuries:

- Changes in consciousness
- Pain along the spine at the site of the injury
- Partial or complete loss of movement in the arms, legs, hands, or feet
- Tingling or loss of sensation in the arms, legs, hands, or feet
- Disorientation
- Abnormal shape of the back or neck
- Bruise(s) over the spine
- Difficulty breathing or no breathing
- Obvious head injury
- Fluid (other than water) or blood in the ears
- Sudden memory loss

Caring for Possible Head, Neck, or Back Injury
In shallow water, follow these steps:

1. Be sure someone has called 9-1-1 or the local emergency number. If other people are present, ask someone to help you.

2. Prevent movement of the victim's head, neck, and back. Try to keep the victim's head in line with the body, but do not pull on the head. Use one of the two methods described in the next section.

3. Position the victim faceup at the surface of the water using the **head splint** method described in the next section. Keep the victim's face out of the water to allow him or her to breathe.

4. Check for consciousness and breathing once you have stabilized the victim's head, neck, and back. A person who can talk is conscious and breathing. If the victim is unconscious and not breathing, remove the victim from the water immediately and provide **rescue breathing**. Attempt to minimize movement of the head, neck, and back when removing the victim from the water. When providing rescue breathing, lift the victim's chin without tilting the head back (jaw thrust) (Fig. 3-21).

5. If the victim is breathing, support the victim in the water with his or her head, neck, and back immobilized until help arrives.

Figure 3-21

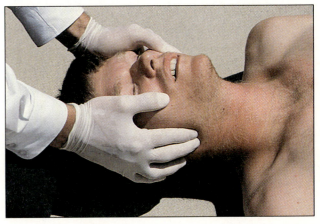

SMALL CRAFT SAFETY

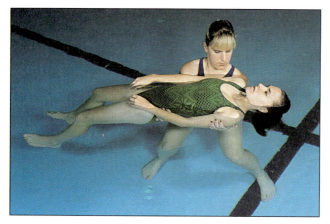

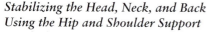

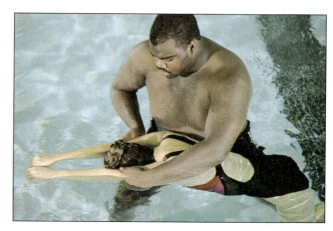

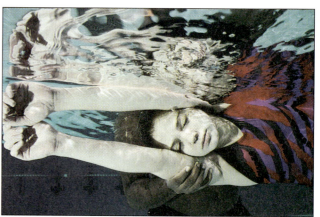

*Stabilizing the Head, Neck, and Back
Using the Hip and Shoulder Support*
Use the **hip and shoulder support** for a victim who is faceup at or near the surface when you reach him or her.

1. Approach the victim from the side, and lower yourself to about shoulder depth.
2. Slide one arm under the victim's shoulders and the other under the hips. Hold the victim's body horizontally, keeping the victim's face out of the water (Fig. 3-22).
3. Do not lift the victim. Hold him or her still in the water until help arrives and takes over.

*Stabilizing the Head, Neck, and Back
Using the Head Splint*
Use the head splint for a victim found facedown at or near the surface.

1. Approach the victim from the side.
2. Gently move the victim's arms up alongside the head by grasping the victim's arms midway between the shoulder and elbow. Move the victim's right arm with your right hand, and the victim's left arm with your left hand.
3. Squeeze the victim's arms against the head to help keep the head in line with the body (Fig. 3-23, A).
4. Glide the victim forward slowly.
5. Move slowly and rotate the victim toward you until he or she is faceup. To rotate the victim, push the victim's closer arm underwater while pulling the other arm across the surface toward you (Fig. 3-23, B).
6. Position the victim's head in the crook of your arm, keeping the head in line with the body (Fig. 3-23, C). In water with currents, hold the victim's head upstream to keep the body from twisting.
7. Do not lift the victim. Hold him or her still in the water until help arrives and takes over.

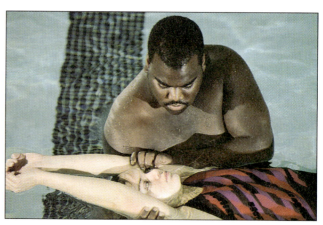

Figure 3-23, A, B and C

Hypothermia

Hypothermia is a life-threatening condition in which the body is unable to maintain warmth and the entire body cools. Hypothermia caused by cold water is especially dangerous. Heat is lost in still water 25 times faster than it is lost in still air of the same temperature. In moving water, the rate of heat loss increases substantially. For instance, in a 5 MPH water current the human body may lose heat 240 times faster than in still air of a similar temperature.

After you enter cold water, several things occur:
- The temperature of your skin and the blood in your arms and legs drops quickly. You may lose the use of your hands.
- Breathing may be hard at first.
- The temperature of your heart, brain, and other vital organs gradually drops.
- Shivering can occur.
- You may become confused and disoriented.
- You may lose consciousness.
- If your temperature continues to drop, heart failure may occur.

The fastest and most common way for death to occur from hypothermia in the water is for the cold water to cause an uncontrollable loss of movement and muscle control. This results in the victim's inability to swim, and eventually leads to drowning.

How Cold Is Cold?

Some define cold water as water that is 70 degrees F or less. Others maintain if it feels cold, then it is cold. Most cases of hypothermia occur when the water temperature is 60 degrees F or less. However, the core temperature begins to drop after a person is exposed to water cooler than 92 degrees for fifteen minutes or longer.[1] It is more important to understand and prevent the potentially deadly effects of cold water than to define cold water. You should recognize the signs of hypothermia, understand some of the factors that affect the onset of hypothermia, and know how to care for it.

[1] USMC, Marine Combat Instructor of Water Survival

PREDICTED SURVIVAL IN COLD WATER

Method	Time (Hrs)
(Without a life jacket)	
Survival floating	1.5
Treading water	2.0
(With a life jacket)	
Swimming	2.0
Holding still	2.7
H.E.L.P. position	4.0
Huddle position	4.0

The survival time is of the average adult in approximately 50° F water

USMC, Marine Combat Instructor of Water Survival

Factors Which Affect Hypothermia Survival

Gender—Women lose heat more slowly than men.
Physical fitness level—The better shape you are in, the better your chances of survival.
Water temperature—The colder the water, the more dangerous it is.
Age—Very old and very young people are more susceptible to hypothermia.
Activity—Remaining motionless in water increases survivability.
Body size—A larger, heavier build increases survival time.
Length of exposure—The longer you are in the water, the less your chances of survival.

USMC, Marine Combat Instructor of Water Survival

Hypothermia Level	Core Body Temperature	Description
Mild (awake with shivers)	99.6	Normal rectal temperature
	96.8	Increased metabolic rate
	95.0	Maximum shivering
	93.2	Victim usually responsive, maximum blood pressure
	91.4	Increasing severity of hypothermia
Moderate	89.6	Consciousness clouded, shivering stops
(awake without shivers)	87.8	Blood pressure difficult to obtain
	86.0	Approaching unconsciousness/rigidity
	85.2	Slow pulse/respiration; cardiac irregularity may develop
Major (unconscious; may	82.4	Ventricular fibrillation may occur
appear to be dead)	80.6	Voluntary motion lost; appears dead
	78.8	Victim seldom conscious
	77.0	Spontaneous ventricular fibrillation
	75.2	Pulmonary edema develops
	71.6	Maximum risk of fibrillation
	69.8	Heart standstill

Source: Smith and Smith, *Water Rescue*, Mosby–Year Book

Protect yourself from hypothermia by—

- Always wearing a U.S. Coast Guard–approved life jacket while boating on cold water. In addition to providing flotation, a life jacket helps conserve body heat.
- Wearing layers of insulated clothes that keep you warm even while wet, such as clothing made from wool or containing polypropylene or capalene.
- Wearing a wet suit or dry suit during aquatic activities.
- Wearing a hat. Body heat is quickly lost through the head.

If you are on a boat and you capsize in cold water—

- Get out of the water, if at all possible.
- Climb up into or onto your boat.
- If other boaters are nearby, signal for them to help you out of the water.
- Do not move around in the water in an attempt to keep warm. This will actually cool your body faster.

Hypothermia is a medical emergency that requires prompt care. Call 9-1-1 or the local emergency number and follow these steps immediately if you fall into cold water.

1. Get out of the water and get to a warm place.
2. Remove wet clothing.
3. Gradually rewarm your body by wrapping yourself in blankets or putting on dry clothes. Cover your head to prevent further heat loss.

Note: Be careful not to rewarm yourself too quickly. Rapid rewarming can cause dangerous heart rhythms.

4. Drink warm nonalcoholic and decaffeinated liquids.

To care for others—

1. Call 9-1-1 or the local emergency number.
2. Get the victim to a warm place.
3. Remove any wet clothing and dry the victim.
4. Gradually rewarm the victim's body by wrapping him or her in blankets or putting dry clothes on the victim. Cover the victim's head to prevent further heat loss.
5. Give warm nonalcoholic and decaffeinated liquids to a conscious victim.
6. For an unconscious victim, monitor the victim's breathing and pulse. Be prepared to give rescue breathing or CPR.

Seizures

You must move quickly to help someone having a **seizure** in the water. A person may suddenly become unconscious and slip underwater without calling for help. He or she may inhale water into his or her lungs, leading to life-threatening conditions. To assist someone having a seizure in the water—

1. Have someone call 9-1-1 or the local emergency number.
2. Support the victim to keep the head and face above water so that he or she can breathe and avoid inhaling water.

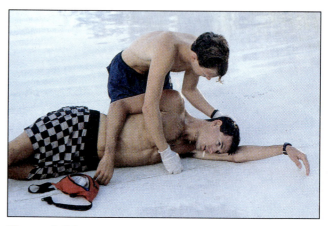

Figure 3-24

3. Remove the victim from the water after the seizure.
4. Place the victim on his or her side to let fluids drain from the mouth (Fig. 3-24).
5. Provide emergency care, if needed (see pages 34-35).

Unconscious Victim

A victim lying motionless and facedown in the water may be unconscious. If the water is not above your chest, wade into the water with flotation equipment. If you do not suspect a head, neck, or back injury, turn the victim face-up, and then bring him or her to the shoreline. Remove the victim from the water and provide emergency care.

If you are boating and must provide care for an unconscious victim, there are several factors you need to consider which may effect the care you provide:

- Weather and water conditions—how deep, shallow, or cold is the water?
- Distance from shore or safety
- Availability of other rescuers
- Type of craft
- Victim's condition

Check the scene and the victim. Consider your own abilities, safety, and available resources.

Emergency Care

The emergency is not over when the victim is out of the water. It is crucial to provide first aid until **EMS personnel** arrive and take over. The care you give can help prevent further injury, disability, or even death. Critical first aid actions include the following:

- If the victim is not breathing, give rescue breathing. If the victim does not have a pulse give CPR (Fig. 3-25).
- If the airway is obstructed, give abdominal thrusts (Heimlich maneuver) for a child or adult, or back blows and chest thrusts for an infant, to clear the airway. Once

CHAPTER **3** *Basic Water Rescue*   35

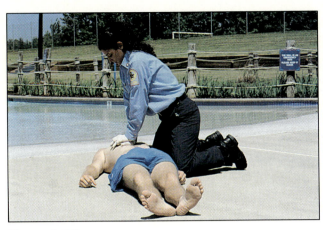

Figure 3-25

the airway is clear, give rescue breathing or CPR, if needed.
- Control bleeding, if necessary.
- If the victim is cold, use dry towels or blankets to keep him or her warm and care for hypothermia.
- If the victim is conscious, reassure and comfort him or her until help arrives.

Note: If you do not have current training in first aid and CPR, contact your local Red Cross for further information about available courses.

SUMMARY

Always wear a life jacket while participating in activities on or around the water. Even if you are a good swimmer, you may find yourself in the water and unable to reach safety. If you do end up in the water, knowing how to stay afloat while awaiting rescue, how to use clothing you may be wearing to help you remain afloat, and how to conserve your body heat can help you to survive.

Helping someone who is having trouble in the water begins with recognizing a distressed swimmer or a drowning victim. You can help a person from the water with a reaching, throwing, wading, or walking assist. Always stay safe when helping a distressed swimmer or drowning victim. Once the person is out of the water, additional emergency care may be needed. If there is a chance the person has a head, neck, or back injury, use special methods to protect the head, neck, or back from further injury. Also, special methods are used for a person who is having a seizure in the water.

Knowing how to perform the techniques described in this chapter may help save a life.

LEARNING ACTIVITIES

TRUE OR FALSE

Circle the correct answer.

1. Screaming or calling for help is the first sign that someone is drowning.   True or False?

2. The safest way to help a person in the water is to go in after him or her.   True or False?

3. With a head, neck, or back injury, your major concerns are to help the person breathe, and prevent the head, neck, or back from moving.   True or False?

4. Heavy winter clothes should be removed as quickly as possible if you fall into cold water.   True or False?

5. Moving around in cold water will help you to keep warm.   True or False?

SMALL CRAFT SAFETY

MULTIPLE CHOICE

Circle the letter of the best answer or answers.

1. Which of the following *does not* characterize an *active drowning* victim?
   a. Arms waving in the air while calling for help
   b. Vertical in the water
   c. Struggles to breathe
   d. Unable to swim
   e. Arms to the sides, alternately moving up and pressing down.

2. After a victim has been pulled from the water—
   a. Give comfort and reassurance.
   b. Check for consciousness and breathing.
   c. Care for hypothermia if the victim is cold.
   d. Check for bleeding and broken bones.
   e. All of the above.

3. If an unconscious person is too heavy for you to carry out of shallow water along the shore, use—
   a. A walking assist.
   b. A wading assist.
   c. A beach drag.
   d. A hip and shoulder support.
   e. A two-person carry.

4. If you fall into warm water while clothed and not wearing a life jacket—
   a. Remove your outer clothing and tread water.
   b. Remove your outer clothing and swim to shore or a dock.
   c. Try to trap air in your clothing and swim or float.
   d. Remove your shoes and swim or float.
   e. None of the above.

5. Prevent hypothermia by—
   a. Treading water to stay warm.
   b. Wearing an approved life jacket when boating on cold water.
   c. Wearing layers of insulated clothes that keep you warm even when wet.
   d. Using caution and wearing a hat when boating on cold water.
   e. Survival floating.

FILL IN

Fill in the correct answers.

1. To rescue a person without entering the water, if possible use a _____ assist. If that does not work, try a _____ assist.

2. Why are seizures a special concern in or around water? _____
_____
_____

3. List at least three situations in which a head, neck, or back injury is possible: _____
_____
_____
_____

4. To stabilize a person in the water who has a suspected head, neck, or back injury, use the _____ _____ for a faceup victim and the _____ for a facedown victim.

5. Describe the two positions for floating in cold water while wearing a life jacket:
HELP (Heat Escape Lessening Posture): _____
_____
_____
_____

Huddle position: _____
_____
_____
_____

CHAPTER 3   Basic Water Rescue

SCENARIOS

1. A friend, whom you know is a poor swimmer, trips on a walkway along a canal and falls into deep water. Panicking, he begins to struggle toward the wall.

   a. What should you do first?
      1. Immediately jump in after him.
      2. Take off your shoes and any heavy clothes, and jump in after him.
      3. Tell him you'll go for help, and quickly seek assistance.
      4. Look for something to reach to him with.
      5. Throw your shirt or jacket to him, and tell him to inflate it.

   b. Name at least two possible objects you could reach to him: _____
      _____
      _____

   c. List the steps for a reaching assist:
      1. _____
      2. _____
      3. _____

   d. If he is too far from the side to reach, what should you do? _____

   e. List at least two possible objects you could throw to him: _____
      _____

   f. Describe the six steps you would follow for a throwing assist:
      1. _____
      2. _____
      3. _____
      4. _____
      5. _____
      6. _____

2. A child playing in the shallow end at the camp's waterfront appears to be having a seizure.

   a. What should you do? _____

   b. After entering the water, what should you do to keep the child from drowning? _____
      _____

   c. After the seizure is over, what should you do?
      _____
      _____

See answers to learning activities on page 83.

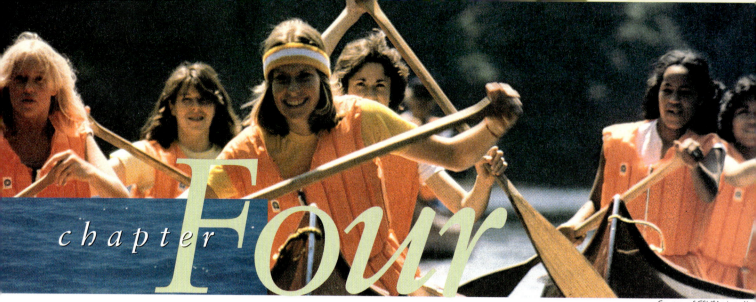

Courtesy of GSUSA photo library

Canoeing Safety

OBJECTIVES

After reading this chapter you should be able to—
1. Identify the parts of a canoe.
2. List the most common causes of canoe accidents, injuries, and fatalities.
3. Explain how to prevent canoe accidents, injuries, and fatalities.
4. Identify and explain the guidelines for safe canoeing.
5. Identify and explain the two rescue priorities of a canoeing emergency.
6. Explain what to do if you fall overboard, capsize, or swamp your canoe in flat water.
7. Explain how to assist others in flat water.
8. Define the key term for this chapter.

After reading this chapter and completing the appropriate course activities, you should be able to—
1. Demonstrate how to reenter your canoe if you fall overboard into flat water.
2. Demonstrate how to rescue yourself if your canoe **swamps** or capsizes.
3. Demonstrate a towing assist on flat water.
4. Demonstrate a canoe-over-canoe rescue.

KEY TERM

Flat water: Lake water or river current where no rapids exist and eddies are slight.

CHAPTER 4 *Canoeing Safety*

INTRODUCTION

Canoeing is a popular activity in the United States. Many people enjoy canoeing as a recreational activity, while others canoe for competition and sport. With a growing number of people in canoes on our waterways, there is an increased need for canoeing safety and education. This chapter discusses the basics of canoeing safety, and what to do if a problem occurs on the water.

THE CANOE

Canoes are made of wood, aluminum, plastic, fiberglass, Kevlar, and other synthetic and natural materials. Despite the variety of canoe types (Fig. 4-1), they have certain common characteristics. You should know some basic terms to understand canoes and canoeing safety.

Bow—The front of a craft.
Gunwale—The top edge of the sides of a craft.
Hull—The main body of a craft.
Painter—A line attached to the bow and/or stern of a craft.
Stern—The back of a craft.
Thwarts (stern, center, and bow)—Support braces in a canoe that go from gunwale to gunwale.

Learning Activity

Using the above terms, complete the following canoe illustration (Fig. 4-2).

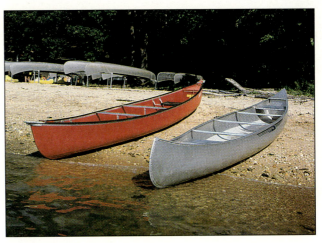

Figure 4-1

CANOEING SAFETY

To understand canoeing safety and prevent canoeing accidents, injuries, and fatalities, you must understand the causes. According to the American Canoe Association, most accidents occur on calm rivers and lakes—not on white water. Approximately half of the canoeing fatalities would not have occurred if the victim had been wearing a life jacket. The effects of alcohol and cold water are also major factors in canoeing accidents and fatalities.[1]

---

[1]C. Walbridge, *River Safety Anthology,* American Canoe Association.

Figure 4-2

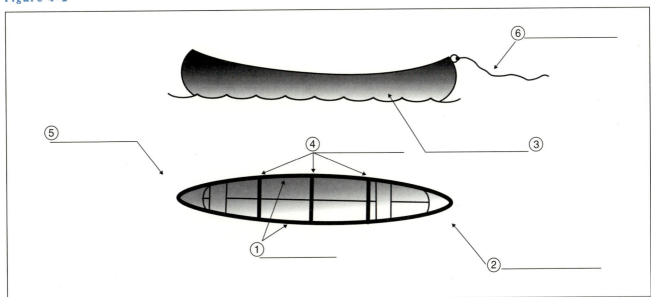

Common canoeing injuries include ankle sprains from walking in or around the water, shoulder injuries from paddling, and back injuries from heavy lifting.[2]

Preventing Canoe Capsizes, Falls Overboard, and Collisions

Capsizes, falls overboard, and collisions are the most common types of canoeing accidents.[3] Most accidents can be prevented by following a few safety guidelines:

- Keep your weight low by paddling in the kneeling position. Passengers should sit on the bottom of the canoe.
- When entering, exiting, or moving around in a canoe, have two hands and one foot, or one hand and two feet in contact with the craft.
- Do not sit on the gunwale.
- Watch out for submerged objects, potential hazards, and other boats.

Guidelines for Safe Canoeing

Understanding the primary causes of canoeing accidents, injuries, and fatalities is the first step to preventing them. The following are important guidelines to provide for your safety and the safety of others while canoeing.

- Canoe in groups. The American Canoe Association recommends there be a minimum of three craft when paddling.
- Have the proper training and experience before supervising others canoeing. This may include training in first aid, CPR, and water safety through your local Red Cross, and training in canoeing through the American Canoe Association, your local Red Cross, and other organizations.
- Make sure everyone on board is wearing a U.S. Coast Guard-approved life jacket.
- Have and use the appropriate clothing, equipment, and gear.
- Check the weather and water conditions before and while canoeing.
- Communicate your expectations, rules, and safety procedures to everyone in the group.
- Be prepared for emergencies, and practice emergency procedures regularly.
- Properly **outfit** the canoe. Attach lines for passengers to hold on to and, if needed, install flotation material to keep the craft afloat if the canoe capsizes or swamps.

- Securely fasten all gear, equipment, and lines to prevent entanglement if the canoe capsizes.
- Do not compromise your safety or the safety of others on the water. Canoe only on waters that are within your ability and within the abilities of others in your group.

SUPERVISION AND COMMUNICATION

Paddlers in the same or different canoes must be able to communicate. In addition to using whistle and hand signals set up in advance, the American Whitewater Affiliation (AWA) has a standardized set of signals to indicate an emergency, get another paddler's attention, and to indicate direction of travel (see Chapter 8, pages 70-71).

Communication between the stern paddler and bow paddler is essential when paddling **tandem**. Clearly communicating basic directions, such as "Forward now!" or "Ready!", can mean the difference between a safe transition through water and an unfortunate mishap.

A canoe trip leader or assistant should make sure that the canoes stay a safe distance apart.

- Each canoe should be within shouting distance of at least one other craft.
- Each canoe should not lose sight of the canoe in front or behind it.
- No canoe should pass the lead canoe or fall behind the sweep canoe.

CANOEING EMERGENCIES

Rescue Priorities

Whenever you are on the water, you should know how to rescue yourself and how to rescue others in an emergency. If a canoeing emergency occurs, follow these rescue priorities:

1. Rescue people first. Your main concern is the health and safety of everyone in your group.
2. After everyone involved has been brought to safety, consider retrieving the craft and gear only if it will not put you or others in danger.

Canoeing Emergencies in Flat Water

Self-Rescue in Flat Water
If you fall overboard in **flat water**, stay with your canoe. Most canoes float and can be used for support. Climbing inside or on top of the canoe will keep you warmer and make you more visible to rescuers.

---

[2] E. Weiss, *Wilderness Medicine*, Mosby–Year Book.
[3] *Boating Statistics 1995* (U.S. Dept. of Transportation, U.S. Coast Guard), September 1995.

CHAPTER 4 *Canoeing Safety*

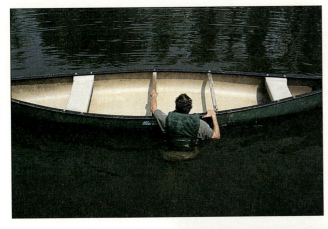
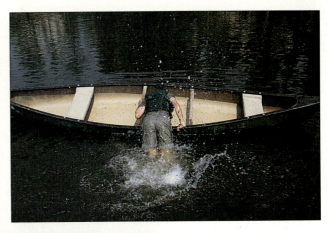
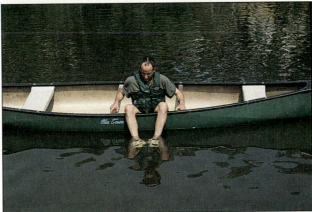

Figure 4-3, A, B and C

Falling Overboard in Flat Water
If you fall overboard:

1. From the side of the canoe, hold on to the gunwale with one hand and a thwart with the other hand (Fig. 4-3, A).
2. Keeping your weight on the gunwale and thwart, kick vigorously to raise your hips to the gunwale (Fig. 4-3, B).
3. Rotate your hips to sit inside the canoe (Fig. 4-3, C), then bring your legs into the craft.
4. If you have a partner, carefully maintain your balance and steady the craft while he or she enters the canoe using the same steps.

Swamped Canoe in Flat Water
If your canoe is swamped but still upright—

1. Turn your canoe toward shore. This will make it easier for you to hand paddle to shore.
2. Lie across the middle of the canoe to keep it from rolling over sideways (Fig. 4-4, A).
3. When the canoe is stable, rotate your body into the canoe (Fig. 4-4, B).
4. Move into a sitting position on the bottom of the craft and hand paddle to safety (Fig. 4-4, C).

5. If you have a partner, carefully steady the craft while he or she enters the canoe using the same steps listed above, then hand paddle to safety.
6. After reaching shallow water empty the water from your canoe.

   1. One paddler stands at the bow while the other paddler stands at the stern (Fig. 4-5, A).
   2. Both paddlers turn the swamped canoe sideways in the water (Fig. 4-5, B).
   3. Lift the canoe sideways out of the water, and empty the canoe (Fig. 4-5, C).
   4. Turn the canoe right-side up, and set it down on the water or carry it ashore.

Assisting Others in Flat Water
Towing Assist
If a canoer has capsized and is close to shore, you can tow the person and their swamped craft to shore. Present the stern of your canoe so that the paddler can hold the painter or the back of your craft (Fig. 4-6). Slowly paddle the person to safety.

Small Craft Safety

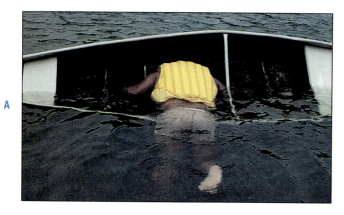
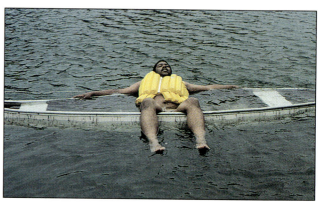
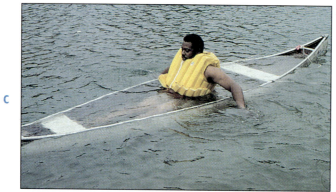

Figure 4-4, A, B and C

Figure 4-5, A, B and C

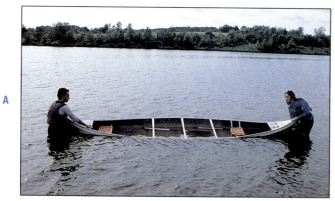
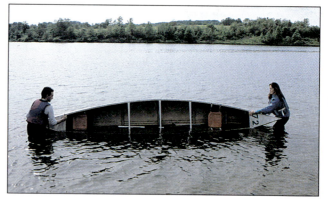
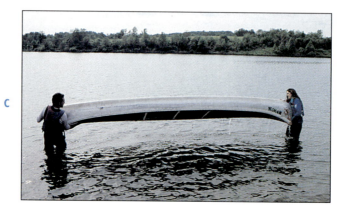

CHAPTER 4 *Canoeing Safety* 43

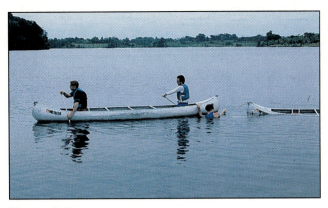
Figure 4-6

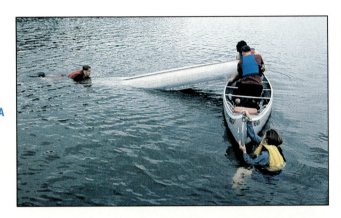
A

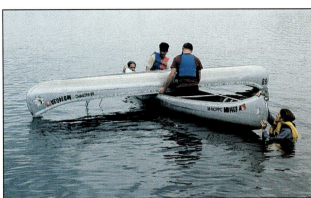
B

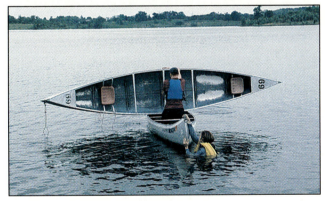
C

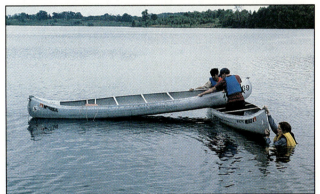
D

Figure 4-7, A, B, C and D

Canoe-over-Canoe Rescue

The canoe-over-canoe rescue is used to empty water from a swamped canoe some distance from shore. During the assist, the capsized paddlers can hold on to each end of your canoe to stabilize it, or one of the capsized paddlers can aid in the assist.

1. The person at the bow of the rescue canoe turns to face the stern.
2. Roll the swamped canoe over so the bottom is up and position it perpendicular to your craft.
3. Lift one end of the upside-down canoe onto the gunwale, near the middle of your canoe (Fig. 4-7, A). At the same time, one of the paddlers in the water pushes down on the end of the canoe that is in the water.
4. Carefully slide the upside-down canoe across the gunwales of your craft (Fig. 4-7, B).
5. Roll the canoe upright while still across the gunwales (Fig. 4-7, C).
6. Slide the canoe back into the water (Fig. 4-7, D). The paddlers can then reenter their canoe while you hold the two canoes side by side for stability.

SUMMARY

Safe canoeing involves understanding the common causes of canoeing accidents, injuries, and fatalities, and knowing how to prevent them. Paddlers also need to know how to communicate with each other when canoeing. Group leaders and individual paddlers must be prepared to act if problems occur while canoeing. This includes knowing the specific techniques for self-rescue and assisting others, and being able to act immediately when a problem begins to develop.

LEARNING ACTIVITIES

TRUE OR FALSE

1. Sitting on the gunwale of the canoe can help prevent capsizing.   True or False?

2. Canoe only on waters that are within your ability and beyond the abilities of others in your group.   True or False?

3. The simple practice of wearing life jackets could prevent half of all canoeing fatalities.   True or False?

MULTIPLE CHOICE

Circle the letter of the best answer or answers.

1. Key strategies for preventing canoeing fatalities include—
    a. Not drinking alcohol while canoeing.
    b. Knowing how to swim.
    c. Wearing a life jacket.
    d. All of the above.

2. Most accidents in canoes occur—
    a. On the ocean.
    b. During storms.
    c. On calm rivers and lakes.
    d. On moving water.

3. When canoeing with other craft, you can help keep the trip safe and enjoyable by—
    a. Staying within sight of the craft immediately in front of and/or behind you.
    b. Staying within shouting distance of at least one other craft.
    c. Staying behind the sweep craft and in front of the lead craft.
    d. Leaving enough space between each craft to avoid collisions.
    e. Leaving a copy of your incident report with the Coast Guard or other authorities.

FILL IN

Fill in the correct answers.

1. The gunwale-to-gunwale braces in a canoe are called _____ .

2. List at least two ways to prevent capsizes, falls overboard, and collisions: _____
_____
_____

3. List the rescue priorities if a canoeing emergency occurs.
    1. _____
    2. _____

4. When attempting a canoe-over-canoe rescue in flat water, why should the capsized paddlers hold onto each end of your craft? _____
_____

CHAPTER 4   *Canoeing Safety*   45

SCENARIOS

1. You are paddling tandem in a canoe across a calm lake to a favorite picnic spot. Without thinking, you stand up to adjust your life jacket. Suddenly you lose your balance, and both you and your canoeing partner fall overboard.

   a. Do you try to get back into the canoe? _____
   b. What caused you to fall out of the canoe?
   _____
   _____

   c. Was this accident preventable?
   _____

   d. Give the four steps to reentering the canoe:
   1. _____
   _____
   2. _____
   _____
   3. _____
   _____
   4. _____
   _____

2. You are paddling across a wide lake with a camp group when one of the canoes capsizes and swamps. After you rescue the canoeists, what are the five steps you take to empty the water from the capsized canoe? You are too far from shore to tow the canoe.

   1. _____
   _____
   2. _____
   _____
   3. _____
   _____
   4. _____
   _____
   5. _____
   _____

See answers to learning activities on pages 83-84.

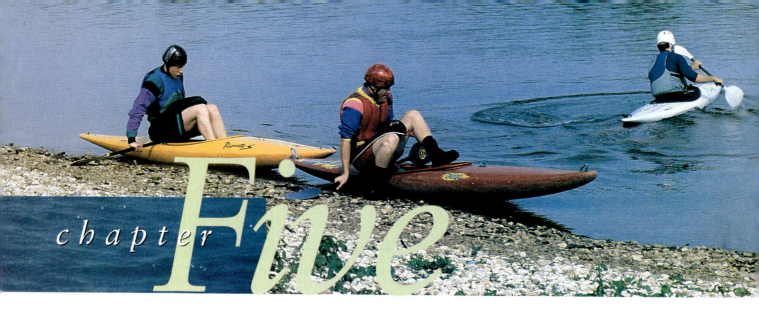

chapter Five

Kayaking Safety

OBJECTIVES

After reading this chapter you should be able to—
1. Identify the different parts of a kayak.
2. Explain how to prevent kayaking accidents, injuries, and fatalities.
3. Identify and explain the guidelines for safe kayaking.
4. Identify and explain the two rescue priorities of a kayaking emergency.
5. Explain what to do if you capsize on flat water.
6. Explain how to assist a capsized paddler from your kayak.
7. Define the key term for this chapter.

After reading this chapter and completing the appropriate course activities, you should be able to—
1. Demonstrate how to wet exit from a capsized kayak.
2. Demonstrate a towing assist with a kayak.
3. Demonstrate a kayak-over-kayak rescue.

KEY TERM

Wet exit: A self-rescue method of exiting a capsized kayak.

CHAPTER 5 *Kayaking Safety*   47

INTRODUCTION

Kayaking has become increasingly popular in recent years. Kayaks are used for recreation, touring, competition, and sport. As with other small craft, the increasing number of kayaks on our waterways increases the need for kayaking safety and education. This chapter discusses the basics of kayaking safety and what to do if a problem occurs on the water.

THE KAYAK

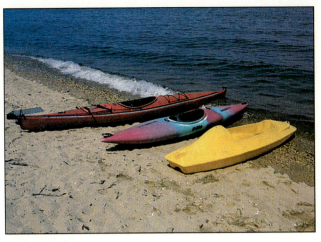

Figure 5-1

Advances in technology and the growing interest in kayaking have led to a wide variety of kayak designs, shapes, and sizes (Fig. 5-1).

Kayaks are often referred to as decked or closed craft because the interior of most kayaks is enclosed, with an opening in the center for the paddler. Kayaks are made of wood, canvas over wood, plastic, fiberglass, Kevlar, and other synthetic or natural materials. The kayak is a unique type of craft that requires specialized skills, distinctive from those needed for other small craft. Despite the various types of kayaks, they have certain characteristics in common. The following are basic terms you need to know to understand kayaks and kayaking safety:

Air bags—Flotation materials placed inside a kayak to provide buoyancy for the craft.
Bow—The front of a craft.
Coaming—A raised rim around the cockpit to which the spray skirt is attached.
Cockpit—The opening in a kayak where the paddler sits.
Deck—The covering over the hull that encloses the interior space.
Grab loop—A coil of line connected to the stern and/or bow of a kayak that is used to grab the craft.
Stern—The back of a craft.

Learning Activity

Using the above terms, complete the following kayak illustration (Fig. 5-2).

KAYAKING SAFETY

To understand kayaking safety and prevent accidents, injuries, and fatalities, you need to understand their causes. Moving water, cold water, and failure to wear life jackets contribute to most kayaking accidents and fatalities.

Figure 5-2

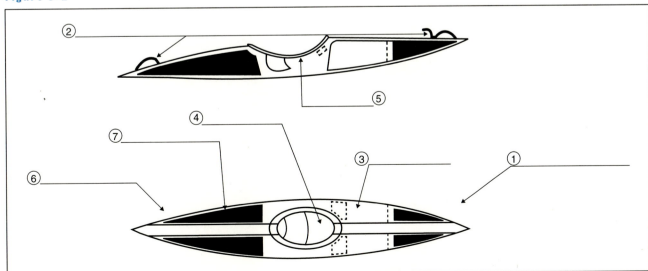

The primary moving-water hazards include long swims, strainers, entrapment in a broached or pinned craft, and hydraulics. Appendix A describes common river hazards. Common injuries include ankle sprains from walking in or around the water, shoulder injuries from paddling, and back injuries from heavy lifting.[1]

Guidelines for Safe Kayaking

The following are important guidelines to provide for your safety and the safety of others while kayaking.

- Learn how to kayak properly.
- Kayak in groups. The American Canoe Association recommends a minimum of three craft when paddling.
- Have the proper training and experience before supervising others kayaking. This may include training in first aid, CPR, and water safety through your local Red Cross, and training in kayaking through the American Canoe Association, your local Red Cross, and other organizations.
- Make sure paddlers wear a U.S. Coast Guard-approved life jacket and an appropriate safety helmet.
- Have and use the appropriate clothing, equipment, and gear.
- Check the weather and water conditions before and while kayaking.
- Communicate your expectations, rules, and safety procedures to everyone in the group.
- Be prepared for emergencies, and practice emergency procedures regularly.
- Properly outfit the kayak. Furnish the craft with safety equipment, provisions, and gear. If flotation is not already installed, install **air bags** to keep the craft afloat in case the kayak capsizes or swamps.
- Securely fasten all gear, equipment, and lines to prevent entanglement if the kayak capsizes.
- Do not compromise your safety or the safety of others on the water. Kayak only on waters that are within your ability and within the abilities of others in your group.

SUPERVISION AND COMMUNICATION

Kayakers need to be able to communicate over the sound of the water, and at a distance. In addition to using whistle and hand signals set up in advance, the American Whitewater Affiliation has a standardized set of signals to indicate an emergency, get another paddler's attention, and to indicate direction of travel (see Chapter 8, pages 70-71).

A kayak trip leader or assistant should make sure that the kayaks stay a safe distance apart.

- Each kayaker should stay within shouting distance of at least one other craft.
- Each kayaker should not lose sight of the kayak in front of or behind it.
- No kayaker should pass the lead kayak or fall behind the sweep kayak.

KAYAKING EMERGENCIES

Rescue Priorities

Whenever you are on the water, be prepared to rescue yourself and know how to rescue others in a kayaking emergency. If a kayaking emergency occurs, follow these rescue priorities:

1. Rescue people first. Your main concern is the health and safety of everyone in your group.
2. After everyone involved has been brought to safety, consider retrieving the craft and gear only if it will not put you or others in danger.

Kayaking Emergencies in Flat Water

Methods of self-rescue depend on whether you are in flat water or moving water.

Self-Rescue in Flat Water

If your kayak capsizes on flat water, stay with your kayak (Fig. 5-3). The kayak will most likely float and support you. Rescuers will also be able to spot you more easily.

Wet Exit in Flat Water

The most common mishap in a kayak is capsizing. If your kayak capsizes, it is easy to get out if you move *slowly and deliberately.* Remember to tuck forward as it capsizes. This will help protect your head.

To exit from a capsized kayak, perform a *wet exit:*

1. Release the **spray skirt** from the coaming (Fig. 5-4, A).
2. With both hands on the side of the craft push yourself out of the kayak (Fig. 5-4, B).
3. Tuck your body forward and pull your legs out together (Fig. 5-4, C).
4. Surface, hold on to the **grab loop**, and swim with it to shore.

Leave the kayak upside down when you swim with it to shore. The air trapped inside the craft makes it buoyant and easier to move.

Once ashore, you can empty the water by raising and lowering one end of the kayak.

---

[1] E. Weiss, *Wilderness Medicine,* Mosby–Year Book.

CHAPTER 5   *Kayaking Safety*   49

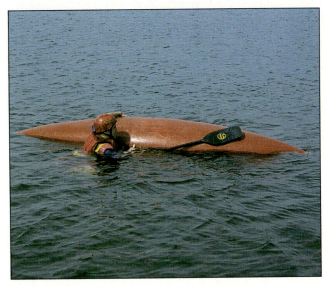

Figure 5-3

Figure 5-4, A, B and C

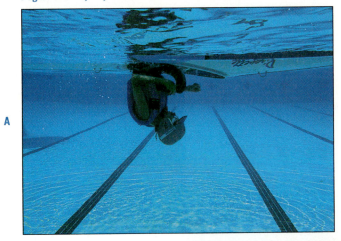

A

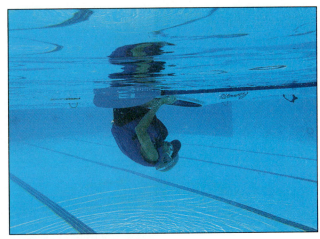

B

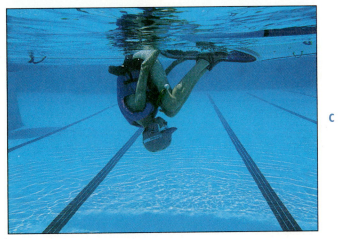

C

50 SMALL CRAFT SAFETY

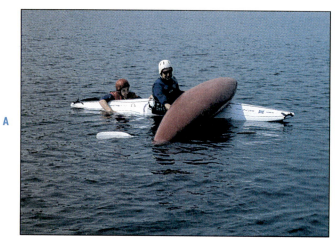

Figure 5-5

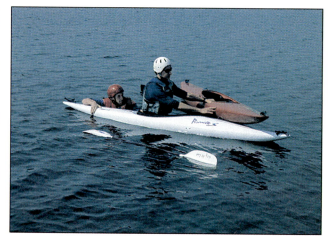

Figure 5-6, A and B

Assisting Others in Flat Water

Towing Assist

If a kayaker capsizes close to shore, you can tow the person and craft back to safety with your kayak. Present the stern of your kayak so that the paddler can hold the stern grab loop of your craft. Have the person hold on to the grab loop of his or her craft. Leave the kayak upside down since the trapped air inside makes it more buoyant. Slowly tow the person and craft to shore (Fig. 5-5).

The Kayak-over-Kayak Rescue

The kayak-over-kayak rescue is used to empty water from a swamped kayak some distance from shore.

1. Have the paddler of the swamped kayak hold on to the stern of your craft to help stabilize it.
2. From your craft, turn the swamped kayak upside down in the water.
3. Pull the upside-down kayak onto your deck (Fig. 5-6, A).
4. Balance the upside-down kayak across your deck, and rock it from one end to the other to empty the water out of the cockpit.
5. Lean your craft from side to side to assist the rocking motion.
6. Once the kayak is empty of water, roll it upright and slide it back into the water (Fig. 5-6, B).
7. Assist the person into their kayak by bracing it alongside yours with the paddles across both craft. Have the person climb on board as you continue to stabilize the craft.

CHAPTER 5 *Kayaking Safety*

SUMMARY

Safe kayaking involves understanding the common causes of kayaking accidents, injuries, and fatalities, and knowing how to prevent them. Kayakers also need to know how to communicate with each other on the water. Trip leaders and individual kayakers must understand the specific kayaking hazards and be prepared to act if a problem occurs. This includes the specific techniques for self-rescue and assisting others in situations that may occur on the water.

LEARNING ACTIVITIES

TRUE OR FALSE

1. Since most kayaks hold only one person, it is recommended that you paddle alone on flat water. True or False?

2. Moving water, cold water, and not wearing life jackets are the most common factors in kayaking accidents and fatalities. True or False?

3. Before swimming your kayak to shore after a capsize, you should turn it right-side up. True or False?

4. A good kayaking leader compromises the safety of the group only if he or she is an experienced paddler. True or False?

MULTIPLE CHOICE

Circle the letter of the best answer or answers.

1. The most frequent mishap in kayaking is—
    a. Losing the paddle in a rapid.
    b. Water entering through the spray skirt.
    c. Capsizing.
    d. Puncturing the hull.

2. Moving water, cold water, and failure to wear life jackets—
    a. Can be avoided by using the kayak-over-kayak rescue.
    b. Contribute to most kayaking accidents and fatalities
    c. Are preventable with proper outfitting.
    d. None of the above.

3. When kayaking with other craft, you can help keep the outing safe and enjoyable by—
    a. Staying within sight of the craft immediately in front of and/or behind you.
    b. Keeping within shouting distance of at least one other craft.
    c. Staying behind the lead craft and in front of the sweep craft.
    d. Leaving enough space between craft to avoid collisions.
    e. All of the above.

4. Which of the following guidelines help to provide for your safety and the safety of others while kayaking?
    a. Have and use the appropriate clothing, equipment, and gear.
    b. Check the weather and water conditions after kayaking.
    c. Communicate your expectations, rules, and safety procedures to everyone in the group.
    d. Be prepared for emergencies, and practice emergency procedures.
    e. Properly outfit the kayak. Furnish the craft with safety equipment, provisions, and gear. If needed, install air bags to keep the craft afloat in case the kayak capsizes or swamps.
    f. Ensure that all gear, equipment, and lines are unfastened and loose to prevent entanglement if the kayak capsizes.

SMALL CRAFT SAFETY

FILL IN

Fill in the correct answers.

1. If your kayak capsizes, you can get out easily if you move _____ and _____ .

2. In addition to a life jacket, kayakers should also wear a _____ .

3. List the two rescue priorities after a kayaking accident:
   1. _____
   2. _____

4. Explain how to assist someone who is in the water close to shore: _____
_____
_____

SCENARIOS

1. You are paddling your kayak on the bay. Suddenly the wake from a passing boat causes you to lose your balance and capsize.

   a. What can you do? _____
   b. What are the four steps to exit a kayak?
      1. _____
      2. _____
      3. _____
      4. _____

2. You are taking some novice kayakers on a wide lake when suddenly one of the kayaks capsizes. After the capsized paddler exits the kayak, he finds that it has taken on a considerable amount of water. What steps should you take to empty water from the swamped kayak?

   1. _____
   2. _____
   3. _____
   4. _____
   5. _____
   6. _____
   7. _____

See answers to learning activities on page 84.

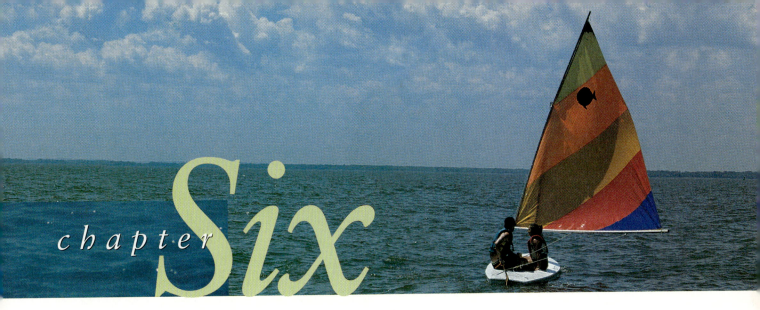

chapter Six

Sailing Safety

OBJECTIVES

After reading this chapter you should be able to—
1. Identify the different parts of a sailboat.
2. List the most common causes of sailing accidents, injuries, and fatalities.
3. Explain how to prevent sailing accidents, injuries, and fatalities.
4. Identify and explain the rules of the road used by sailors.
5. Identify and explain standard communication signals for sailors.
6. Identify and explain the two rescue priorities of a sailing emergency.
7. Explain what to do if your sailboat capsizes.
8. Explain how to assist a sailor who has fallen overboard.
9. Define the key terms for this chapter.

After reading this chapter and completing the appropriate activities, you should be able to—
1. Demonstrate a capsize recovery for one sailor.
2. Demonstrate a scoop recovery.
3. Demonstrate an overboard recovery.

KEY TERMS

Heel: When a boat leans over to one side because of the pressure of wind on the sail(s).
Jibe: To change from one tack to another when sailing downwind.
Rigging: The lines and fittings used to adjust the sails.

Safety position: When a boat is stopped with its sails eased and flapping, and the wind coming from the side.
Tack: The orientation of a boat based on the side of the boat nearer the wind (i.e., a starboard tack or port tack). Also, to change from one tack to another when sailing upwind.

INTRODUCTION

Every year many people enjoy sailing. Sailing for recreation, cruising, or sport is exhilarating and fun. With a large number of sailboats and other craft on our waterways, there is an increased need for sailing safety and education. This chapter discusses the basics of sailing safety and what to do if a problem occurs on the water.

THE SAILBOAT

There are numerous types, shapes, and sizes of sailboats (Fig. 6-1). Despite the various types of sailboats, they have certain characteristics in common. Following are some basic terms you need to know to understand sailboats and sailing safety:

Boom—A wooden or metal pole attached to the mast that holds out the bottom of a sail.
Bow—The front of a craft.
Centerboard—An inserted or pivoting plate of wood, fiberglass, or metal that projects below the bottom of a sailboat to help prevent the boat from sliding sideways due to the wind. Some types of centerboards are also called daggerboards.
Gunwale—The top edge of the sides of a craft.
Hull—The main body of a craft.
Main sheet—The line used to pull in or let out a **mainsail**.
Mast—The vertical wooden or metal pole in a sailboat that holds up the sail.
Port—The left side of a craft.
Rudder—A flat, vertical plate that is used to steer the boat.
Starboard—The right side of a craft.
Stern—The back of a craft.
Tiller—The handle attached to the top of a rudder used to steer a craft.

Learning Activity

Using the above terms, complete the sailboat illustration on page 55 (Fig. 6-2).

SAILING SAFETY

Safety factors are somewhat different for sailboats than for other small craft. Because they are powered by the wind, and the wind is difficult to control, sailboats have unique operating and safety considerations. To understand sailing safety and prevent sailing accidents, injuries, and fatalities, you need to understand the common causes of sailing accidents, injuries, and fatalities.

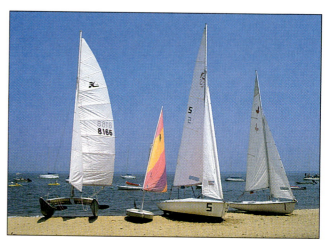

Figure 6-1

Preventing Sailing Accidents, Injuries, and Fatalities

According to the U.S. Coast Guard, most sailing fatalities are a result of drowning. Most sailing accidents occur because of collisions with other vessels, capsizes, and falls overboard.

To prevent sailing accidents, injuries, and fatalities, wear your life jacket, act safely to prevent collisions, and know how to prevent capsizes and falls overboard.

Preventing Collisions

Collisions generally result from carelessness and ignorance of the rules of the road. To prevent collisions, you must look out for other craft and follow the rules of the road. In Chapter 1 you learned some basic rules of the road. Since you may be sailing on busy waters that are shared by many other sailboats, powerboats, and commercial vessels, you need to learn the following additional rules of the road:

- A sailboat on a starboard *tack* has right-of-way over a sailboat on a port tack. That is, a sailboat that has the wind coming across its starboard side has right-of-way over a sailboat that has the wind coming over its port side (Fig. 6-3).
- When two boats are on the same tack, the **leeward** boat has right-of-way over the **windward** boat. The sailboat that is upwind must yield right-of-way (Fig. 6-4).
- Sailboats that are under sail generally have right-of-way over powerboats and sailboats that are motoring. Since most powerboats are faster and more maneuverable than sailboats, they should stay clear of or yield right-of-way to sailboats. The following are exceptions to this rule:
  - Large ocean-going vessels, tugs, barges, and fishing boats pulling nets have right-of-way because of their limited maneuverability and speed.

CHAPTER 6   *Sailing Safety*   55

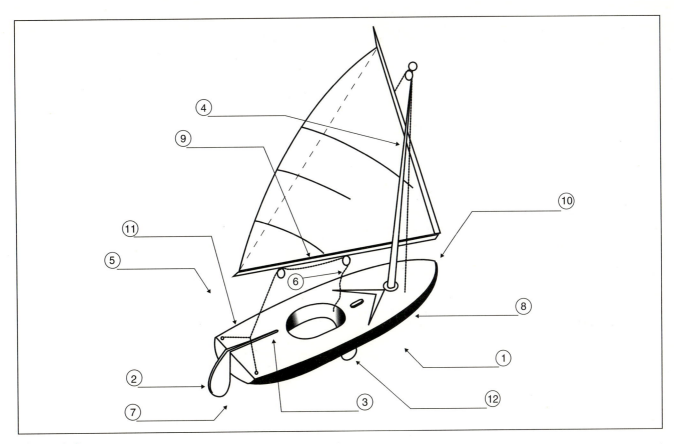

Figure 6-2

Figure 6-3

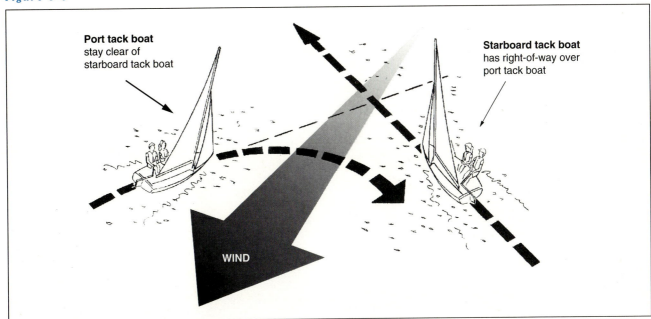

Source: United States Sailing Association, *Start Sailing Right*, 1997. Used with permission.

SMALL CRAFT SAFETY

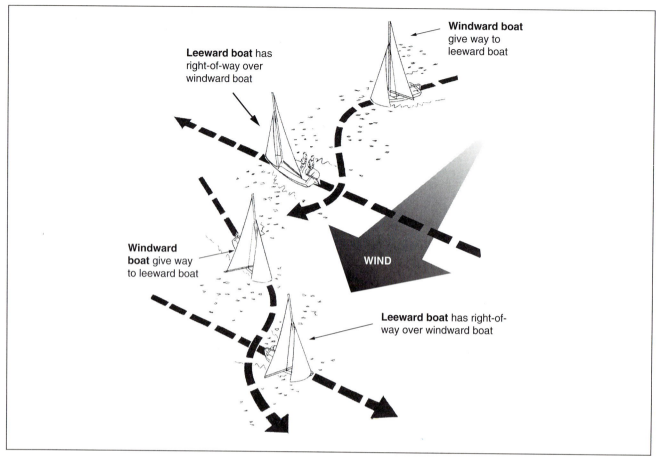

Figure 6-4 — Source: United States Sailing Association, *Start Sailing Right*, 1997. Used with permission.

- Sailboats must also yield right-of-way if overtaking a powerboat.
- Regardless of the type or size of the craft, all boat operators are responsible for avoiding collisions.

For more information on navigational laws and rules of the road, obtain a copy of "Navigation Rules: International-Inland," (COMDTINST M 1667.2B), by contacting Superintendent of Documents, U.S. Government Printing Office, P.O. Box 371954, Pittsburgh, PA 15250-7954, or by contacting your state boating law administrator (Appendix F).

Preventing Capsizes and Falls Overboard

Small sailboats with a centerboard are less stable and more likely to capsize than a sailboat with a **keel**. Those learning to sail should learn what to do and practice how to return a capsized sailboat to an upright position (see page 58).

Some common reasons why small sailboats capsize include the following:

- A sudden gust of wind can catch a sailor by surprise and overpower the boat.
- A poorly executed *jibe* can unbalance the boat and make it suddenly *heel* or tip to one side.
- A broken tiller can cause the operator to lose control.
- Letting go of the tiller or main sheet can cause a sudden change in the angle of heel.
- A quick turn in heavy winds can cause the boat to roll over.[1]

Falls overboard, like most other boating accidents, can be prevented. Use good judgment, learn to sail correctly, and follow these guidelines to prevent falls overboard:

- Maintain control of the sailboat.
- Keep your weight low in the sailboat.
- When entering, exiting, or moving around on a sailboat, have two hands and one foot, or one hand and two feet in contact with the craft.
- Make sure the boat and all of its parts are in good working order.
- Watch for submerged objects, potential hazards, and other boats.
- Communicate to others on board before jibing or turning suddenly.
- Do not sail in heavy winds or thunderstorms.
- Be aware that your head could be struck by the boom if it swings unexpectedly.

---

[1] United States Sailing Association, *Start Sailing Right*, 1997

SUPERVISION AND COMMUNICATION

Sailors on different boats and supervisors in safety boats need to be able to communicate. Since the sounds of water, wind, sails and other noises make it difficult to hear, hand signals are often used. Figures 6-5 to 6-11 show the basic hand signals.

Chapter 2 emphasizes the importance of an adequate number of leaders when boating. You also learned about positioning leaders in boats among participants to make sure that all sailboats can be safely observed. In addition, make sure the sailboats maintain an adequate distance from each other. When sailing or supervising sailors, follow these guidelines:

- Sail in groups.
- Have your group review and practice small craft safety emergency procedures, communication signals, and rules of the road.
- Define the boundaries for how far the sailboats may sail.
- The supervisor of the sailing activity should have documented experience or training for operating the supervisory craft or safety boat.

Figure 6-5

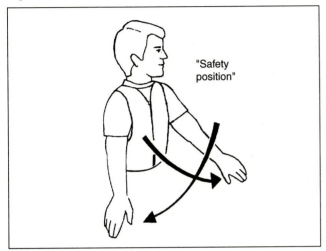

Figure 6-7

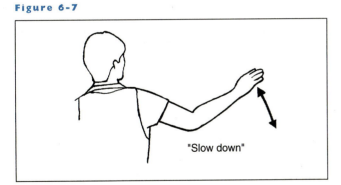

Figure 6-9

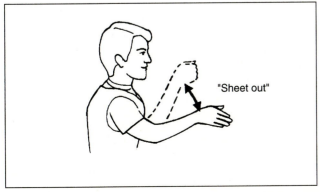

Figure 6-6

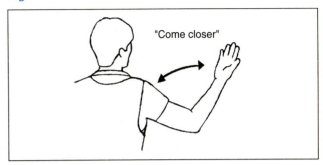

Figure 6-8

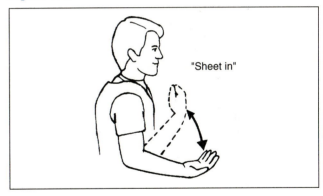

Figure 6-10

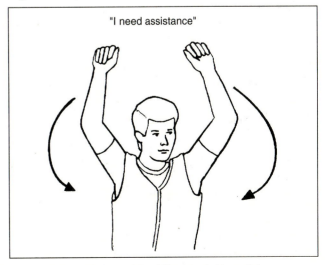

Source: United States Sailing Association, *Start Sailing Right*, 1997. Figures 6-5 to 6-11 reprinted with permission.

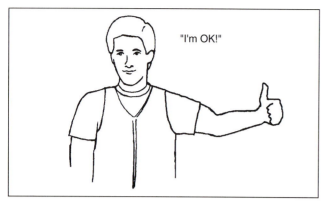

Figure 6-11

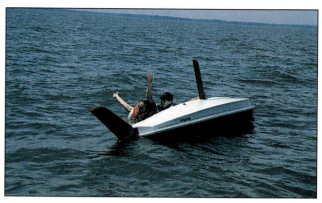

Figure 6-12

SAILING EMERGENCIES

In Chapter 2, you learned about the types of aquatic emergencies and emergency preparation. The best approach to sailing emergencies is to prevent them from happening in the first place. However, no matter how careful and safe you are, emergencies can still happen. Therefore, you should have an emergency action plan and practice it regularly. You also need to know how to rescue yourself and others in the event of a capsize or fall overboard.

Rescue Priorities

Whenever you are on the water, be prepared to rescue yourself or assist others in an emergency. If a sailing emergency occurs, follow these rescue priorities:

1. Rescue people first. Your main concern is the health and safety of everyone in your group.
2. After everyone involved has been brought to safety consider retrieving the craft and gear only if it will not put you or others in danger.

Self-Rescue after Sailboat Capsize

Most centerboard boats are self-rescuing, which means you can right the boat yourself and be sailing again in a few minutes. Self-rescuing boats make capsize recovery easier. (Make sure the drain plugs in air tanks or flotation bags are securely fastened before you go sailing.)

The most common way for a sailboat to capsize is for it to roll over leeward, away from the wind. The sails then usually lie on the water downwind from the boat. Boats can also roll over windward, toward the wind. This happens less frequently, but usually more quickly than a leeward capsize.

If you do capsize and cannot right the sailboat, remember the most important rule: *Stay with the boat.* It should float and support you, and rescuers will be able to spot you more easily. Hold on to the boat or climb up onto the hull and signal for help (Fig. 6-12).

There are different ways you can right a sailboat after a capsize, depending on the size and type of boat, number of crew, and your experience.

Before trying to right the craft, check that—

- Everyone is free of lines, sail, and *rigging*.
- The main sheet is free.
- The rudder and tiller are still attached.
- The centerboard is in the down position.

Capsize Recovery for One Sailor
Use the following method to recover a capsized sailboat by yourself. Be careful when recovering the craft in strong winds. The boat could capsize again because no one else is holding onto the boat to balance it.

1. Rotate the boat so the bow is facing into the wind.
2. Climb onto the centerboard and grab the gunwale. Swing the boat upright (Fig. 6-13). If more weight is needed, carefully stand on the centerboard, hold on to the gunwale, and swing the sailboat upright.
3. Reboard the boat at the stern.

Scoop Recovery
Use this recovery method to scoop one or more capsized sailors into the boat as it is righted:

1. Have the sailor hold on to the inside of the cockpit (Fig. 6-14, A).
2. While holding on to the gunwale and the centerboard, swing the boat upright, scooping the sailor into the cockpit (Fig. 6-14, B). If more leverage is needed, carefully stand on the centerboard, hold on to the gunwale, and swing the sailboat upright.
3. Have the sailors inside the sailboat put the sailboat into the *safety position* while you hold on to the side.
4. Enter the craft at the stern.[2]

---

[2]Ibid.

CHAPTER **6** *Sailing Safety*

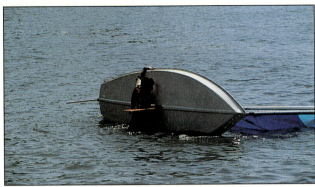

Figure 6-13

Overboard Recovery

Assist someone who has fallen overboard using the overboard recovery.

1. Alert other crew members on board by shouting "crew overboard." Keep the victim in sight and tack as soon as possible.
2. Approach from downwind. This minimizes the danger of hitting the victim with the sailboat as you approach (Fig. 6-15, A).
3. Place your sailboat in the safety position next to the victim (Fig. 6-15, B).
4. Have the victim enter at the stern of the sailboat (Fig. 6-15, C).

Figure 6-14, A and B

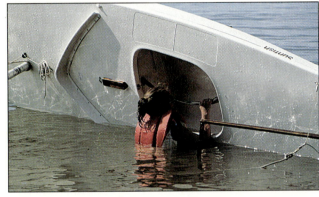 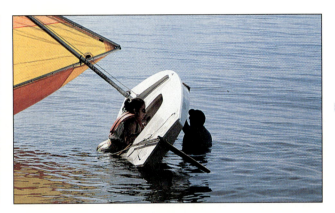

Figure 6-15, A, B and C

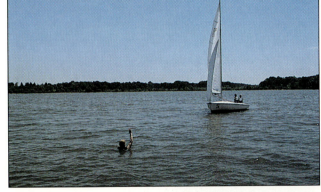 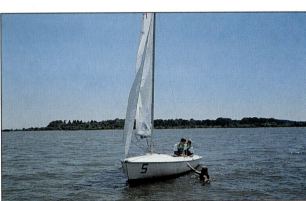

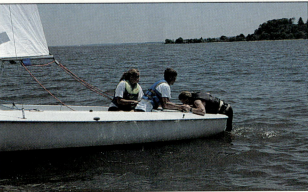

- If the victim needs assistance, reach with a life jacket or other object and pull him or her to the stern of the sailboat.

- If the victim cannot hold onto the life jacket, grasp the victim, pull him or her to the stern, and help the person on board.

SUMMARY

Staying safe while sailing involves understanding the common causes of sailing accidents, injuries, and fatalities, and knowing how to prevent them. Sailors also need to know how to communicate with each other. Trip leaders and individual sailors must understand the particular hazards of sailboats, and be prepared to act if they have a problem on the water. This includes the specific techniques for self-rescue or helping others in any situation that may occur while sailing, such as a capsize or man overboard. The best way to avoid a sailing accident is to prevent it from happening in the first place.

LEARNING ACTIVITIES

TRUE OR FALSE

1. Sailing collisions generally are caused by carelessness or ignorance of the rules of the road. True or False?

2. In an "overboard" emergency, you should immediately drop the mainsail. True or False?

3. The best way to avoid a sailing accident is to prevent it from happening. True or False?

4. Every boat operator is responsible for avoiding collisions—regardless of the type or size of boat. True or False?

MULTIPLE CHOICE

Circle the letter of the best answer or answers.

1. The boom on a sailboat is—
    a. A wooden or metal pole used to attach and hold out the bottom of the sail.
    b. The vertical wooden or metal pole that holds up the sail.
    c. Another name for daggerboard.
    d. The flat, vertical plate used to steer the boat, or rudder.

2. Sailboats generally have right-of-way over which of the following:
    a. Tugboats towing barges
    b. Fishing boats pulling nets
    c. Power boats
    d. Large ocean-going vessels.
    e. None of the above.

3. When two sailboats on different tacks approach each other, the sailboat with right-of-way is—
    a. The sailboat on a port tack.
    b. The sailboat on a starboard tack.
    c. The faster of the two boats.
    d. The larger of the two boats.

4. Sailboats capsize for a number of reasons, including—
    a. Letting go of the tiller or main sheet.
    b. A poorly executed jibe.
    c. A sudden gust of wind.
    d. A fall overboard.

CHAPTER 6 *Sailing Safety*

FILL IN

Fill in the correct answers.

1. List some important safety principles to prevent sailing accidents, injuries, and fatalities—
   _____
   _____
   _____
   _____

2. Collisions generally result from _____ and _____ .

3. If you capsize, and cannot right the craft, the most important rule is to _____ .

4. List the two rescue priorities after any sailing accident.
   1. _____
   2. _____

5. Three common reasons why sailboats capsize include—
   1. _____
   2. _____
   3. _____

SCENARIOS

1. You are sailing solo across a bay in a small, open-cockpit sailboat. The breeze picks up and the boat begins to heel sharply. Instead of easing out the main sheet, you sheet in hard. The boat capsizes.

   a. What is the main thing to remember?
      _____

   b. What are the steps to recover the capsized boat?
      1. _____
      2. _____
      3. _____

   c. If you are unable to recover the boat, what should you do?
      _____

   d. Explain why: _____

2. You are on a sailboat with novice sailors when a sudden tack causes one of the sailors to fall overboard.

   What should you do?
   1. _____
      _____
   2. _____
      _____
   3. _____
      _____
   4. _____
      _____

See answers to learning activities on pages 84-85.

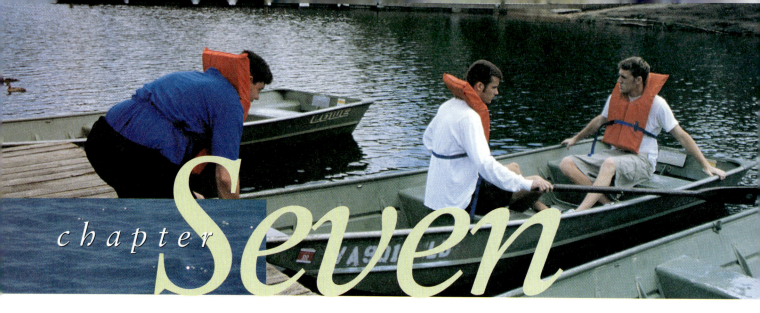

chapter Seven

Rowing Safety

OBJECTIVES

After reading this chapter you should be able to—
1. Identify the different parts of a rowboat.
2. List the most common causes of rowing accidents, injuries, and fatalities.
3. Explain how to prevent most rowing accidents, injuries, and fatalities.
4. Identify and explain the two rescue priorities of a rowing emergency.
5. Explain what to do if your rowboat swamps or you fall overboard.
6. Explain how to assist a victim who has capsized or fallen overboard.
7. Define the key terms for this chapter.

After reading this chapter and completing the appropriate course activities, you should be able to—
1. Demonstrate how to reenter a rowboat from a fall overboard.
2. Demonstrate how to reenter a swamped rowboat.
3. Demonstrate a reaching assist from a rowboat.
4. Demonstrate a throwing assist from a rowboat.

KEY TERMS

Rocker: The curve of the keel from bow to stern. The greater the curve, the less resistance to turning.

Safety boat: A boat used for supervising or recovering other craft, also called a chase boat.

CHAPTER **7** *Rowing Safety*

INTRODUCTION

Whether rowing for exercise or rowing across a calm lake to go fishing, rowboats have always been useful and popular. Different types of rowboats are found on rivers, lakes, the ocean—just about anywhere there is water. With more small craft on our waterways, there is a greater need for boating safety and education. This chapter discusses the basics of rowing safety, and what to do if a problem occurs on the water.

THE ROWBOAT

There are many types, shapes, and sizes of rowboats (Fig. 7-1). A common type of rowboat that is used for recreational activity is the flat-bottom rowboat. It is designed for protected waters and has very little fore (front) and aft (back) *rocker* on the bottom. Despite the various types of rowboats, they have certain characteristics in common. Following are some basic terms you need to know to understand rowboats and rowing safety:

Bow—The front of a craft.
Gunwale—The top edge of the sides of a craft.
Hull—The main body of a craft.
Stern—The back of a craft.
Stern seat—The back seat of a craft.
Transom—The flat, vertical, back end of a rowboat.

Learning Activity

Using the above terms, complete the following rowboat illustration (Fig. 7-2).

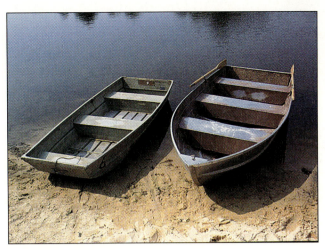

Figure 7-1

ROWING SAFETY

To understand rowing safety and to prevent rowing accidents, injuries, and fatalities, you need to understand their causes. According to the U.S. Coast Guard, most rowing fatalities are a result of drowning. Most rowing accidents involve a capsize or fall overboard.

Preventing Rowing Accidents, Injuries, and Fatalities

The most important safety principles include wearing your life jacket and knowing how to prevent a capsize or fall overboard.

Figure 7-2

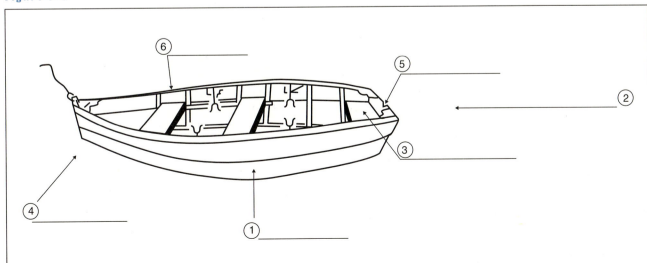

Preventing Capsizes and Falls Overboard

Capsizes and falls overboard, like most other boating accidents, can be prevented. Use good judgment and follow these guidelines to avoid capsizes and falls overboard:

- Keep your weight low in the rowboat.
- When entering, exiting, or moving around in a rowboat, keep two hands and one foot, or one hand and two feet in contact with the craft.
- Do not sit on the gunwale.
- Make sure the rowboat and all of its parts are in good working order.
- Watch for submerged objects, potential hazards, and other boats.
- Do not row in heavy winds, waves, or thunderstorms.

Guidelines for Safe Rowing

The following are important guidelines to provide for your safety and the safety of others while rowing.

- Row in groups.
- Have your group review and practice small craft safety and emergency procedures.
- Review and practice communication signals, including whistle signals and hand signals, with your group.
- Define the boundaries for how far the boats may travel.
- Make sure each rowboat is within shouting distance of at least one other craft.
- The supervisor of the rowing activity should have documented experience or training in operating the supervisory craft or *safety boat*.

ROWING EMERGENCIES

In Chapter 2 you learned about the types of aquatic emergencies and emergency preparation. The best approach to rowing emergencies is to prevent them from happening in the first place. However, no matter how careful and safe you are, emergencies can happen. Therefore, you need to have and practice an emergency action plan. You also need to know how to rescue yourself and others in the event of a rowing emergency.

Rescue Priorities

Whenever you are on the water, be prepared to rescue yourself or assist others in an emergency. In any emergency situation, keep these rescue priorities in mind:

1. Rescue people first. Your main concern is the health and safety of everyone in your group.
2. After everyone involved has been brought to safety, consider retrieving the craft and gear only if it will not put you or others in danger.

Self-Rescue

If your rowboat capsizes or if you fall overboard, stay with your craft. The rowboat will probably float and support you. Rescuers will also be able to spot you more easily.

Self-Rescue from a Fall Overboard

To reenter a rowboat if you have fallen overboard:

1. Place your hands on the transom (Fig. 7-3, A).
2. Kick vigorously and raise your hips while keeping your weight on the transom (Fig. 7-3, B).
3. Rotate your hips and sit on the stern seat, or in the back of the craft.
4. Swing your legs into the rowboat (Fig. 7-3, C).

Self-Rescue from a Capsized or Swamped Rowboat

During a rowboat capsize, you could be struck on the head by the rowboat as it turns over. If your rowboat is capsizing, keep your eyes open, and pay attention to where you are in relation to the boat. Remember the most important rule: *Stay with the boat*. After the capsize, stay calm and hold onto the rowboat. If the boat cannot be righted, hold onto the craft or climb up onto the hull and signal for help. You will be safer with the boat, and rescuers will be able to see you better. If your boat is upright, you can reenter the swamped rowboat and hand paddle to shore.

If your rowboat is swamped—

1. Pull yourself up and over the side at the middle of the boat and lie across it to keep it from rolling side to side (Fig. 7-4, A).
2. Once the boat is stabilized, rotate your body (Fig. 7-4, B).
3. Turn to a sitting position and hand paddle to safety (Fig. 7-4, C), or signal for help.

Rescuing Others from the Water

Use a reaching or throwing assist to help someone who has capsized or fallen overboard.

Reaching Assist

1. Present the stern end of the boat to the victim.
2. From the stern, reach an **oar**, extra life jacket, or other object to the person (Fig. 7-5, A).
3. Pull the person to the stern.
4. Assist the person over the transom into the stern of the craft (Fig. 7-5, B).

Throwing Assist

If you cannot maneuver close to the person, or if the person is too far away for a reaching assist, use a throwing assist. A heaving line, ring buoy, throw bag, rescue tube, or homemade device can be used. Any floating object at hand, such as a buoyant cushion or extra life jacket, can be thrown.

CHAPTER 7   *Rowing Safety*   65

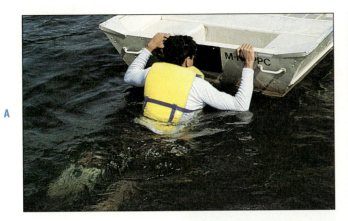
A

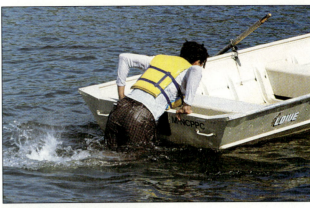
B

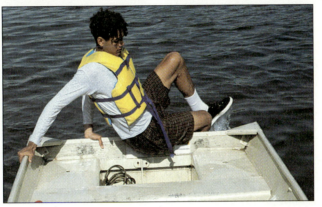
C

Figure 7-3, A, B and C

Figure 7-4, A, B and C

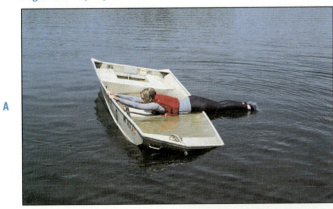
A

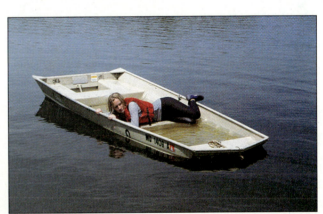
B

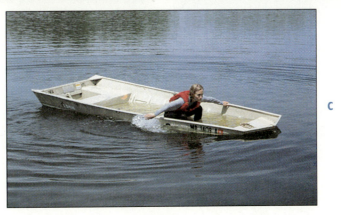
C

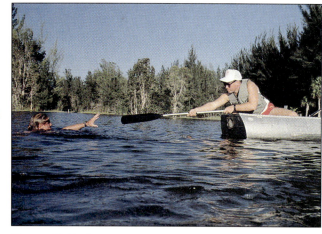
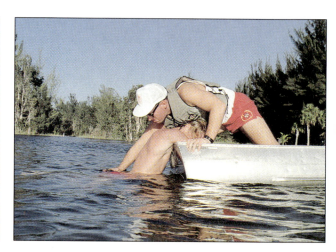

Figure 7-5, A and B

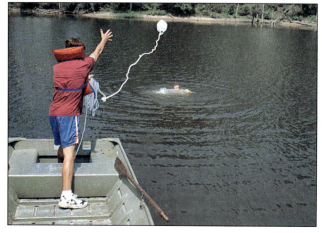
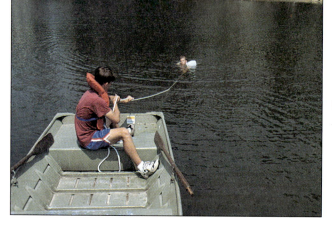

Figure 7-6, A and B

Throwing equipment should be available on small craft and at waterfront areas.

To perform a throwing assist—

1. Get into a stride position: the leg opposite your throwing arm is forward. This helps to keep your balance when you throw the object.
2. Step on the end of the line with your forward foot.
3. Shout to get the victim's attention. Make eye contact and say you are going to throw the object now. Tell the victim to grab it.
4. Bend your knees and throw the object to the victim (Fig. 7-6, A). Try to throw the object upwind and/or current, just over the victim's head, so the line drops within reach.
5. When the victim grasps the object or line, slowly pull him or her to the stern of the craft. Lean away from the water as you pull (Fig. 7-6, B).
6. If the object does not reach the victim, quickly pull the line back in and throw it again. Try to keep the line from tangling, but do not waste time trying to recoil it.
7. Assist the victim over the transom into the stern of the craft.

CHAPTER **7**   *Rowing Safety*   **67**

SUMMARY

The best way to avoid rowing accidents, injuries, and fatalities, is to understand their causes and know how to prevent them. Trip leaders and individual rowers must understand the hazards of rowing and be prepared to act if they have a problem on the water. This includes knowing the specific techniques for self-rescue and assisting others in any situation that may occur, such as falling overboard or capsizing.

LEARNING ACTIVITIES

TRUE OR FALSE

1. The best way to avoid a rowing accident is to prevent it from happening.   True or False?

2. Most rowing fatalities are a result of drowning.   True or False?

3. It is generally safer to row alone.   True or False?

4. Rowboat operators must be prepared to rescue a passenger because most falls overboard cannot be prevented.   True or False?

MULTIPLE CHOICE

Circle the letter of the best answer or answers.

1. Which of the following items is *not* a key strategy for preventing falls overboard while rowing?
    a. Keep your weight low in the rowboat.
    b. When moving around in the rowboat, keep two hands and one foot, or one hand and two feet in contact whith the craft.
    c. Know CPR.
    d. Do not sit on the gunwale.
    e. Watch for submerged objects, potential hazards and other boats.

2. The proper way to approach a person who has fallen overboard in a rowboat is—
    a. With the bow of the boat.
    b. With the side closest to where you are sitting.
    c. With the stern of the boat.
    d. With the gunwale of the boat.

3. Guidelines for safe rowing include—
    a. Review and practice emergency procedures.
    b. Review and practice communications signals.
    c. Define travel boundaries.
    d. a and c, only.
    e. Row in groups.

4. The rescue priorities in a rowboat emergency are—
    a. Craft, people, gear.
    b. Emergency action plan, people, gear.
    c. People, emergency action plan, craft and gear.
    d. People, then craft and gear.

5. Most rowing fatalities are a result of drowning. What single act could have prevented most of these drownings?
    a. If the victims had been wearing life jackets.
    b. If the victims had nighttime visual distress signals.
    c. If the victims had taken most their clothes off and swam for shore.
    d. If the trip leaders had supervised from the lead craft.

SMALL CRAFT SAFETY

FILL IN

Fill in the correct answers.

1. The most important safety principles to prevent rowing accidents, injuries, and fatalities are—
_____
_____
_____

2. If you capsize, the single most important rule is to _____ .

3. Name at least four objects that might be thrown to a person who has fallen overboard.
_____
_____
_____
_____

4. List the two rescue priorities in a rowing accident.
   1. _____
   2. _____

5. If you fall overboard stay with your craft because you will _____, and rescuers _____ .

SCENARIOS

1. You are rowing out to your sailboat when a large wake from a speeding powerboat strikes your rowboat hard on the side, causing you to lose your balance and fall overboard.

   a. What are the steps to reboarding the rowboat?
   _____
   _____
   _____
   _____

   b. If you cannot reboard the boat, what should you do?
   _____

2. While rowing to a favorite fishing spot on a sunny afternoon, one of your two friends stands up to reel in a large fish. He loses his balance, and falls overboard.

   a. What type of assist would be appropriate?
   _____

   b. List the steps.
   1. _____
   2. _____
   3. _____
   4. _____

See answers to learning activities on page 85.

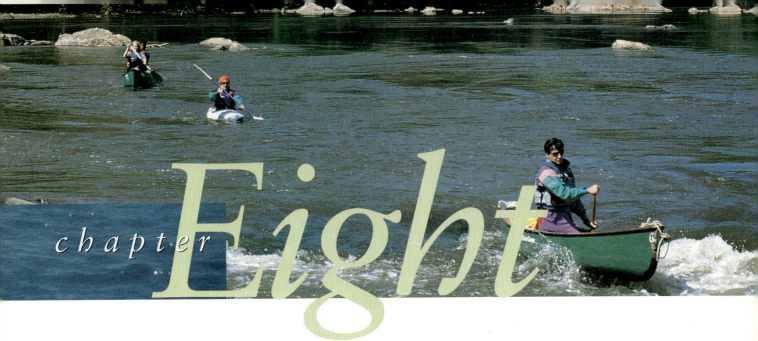

chapter Eight

Moving-Water Safety—Canoeing and Kayaking

OBJECTIVES

After reading this chapter you should be able to—
1. List and describe moving-water hazards.
2. Explain how to prevent moving-water accidents, injuries, and fatalities.
3. Identify the guidelines for moving-water safety.
4. Identify and explain the five American Whitewater Affiliation (AWA) Universal River Signals.
5. Explain how to rescue yourself in moving water.
6. Explain how to assist others in moving water.
7. Define the key terms for this chapter.

After reading this chapter and completing the appropriate course activities, you should be able to—
1. Demonstrate how to float downstream and swim to shore or into an eddy.
2. Demonstrate how to swim over a strainer.
3. Demonstrate a throw bag assist with belay.

KEY TERMS

Eddy: The sheltered area behind or downstream of an obstruction, where the currents flow upstream toward the obstruction.
Entrapment in a canoe or kayak: When the force of the current traps a person between the craft and a rock or obstacle, or collapses the boat and traps a paddler inside the craft.
Foot entrapment: When a person's foot is wedged between or underneath rocks or another submerged object in moving water.
Hole: A type of hydraulic that is formed by a rock, ledge, or other obstruction in a river.

Hydraulic: Strong force created by water flowing downward over an obstruction and then reversing its flow.
Low-head dam: A barrier built across streams and rivers to control the flow of water.
Strainer: An obstacle in a river, often a fallen tree snarled with branches and other debris, that acts like a colander. Water is forced through the obstacle, entrapping or "straining" debris and people.

69

INTRODUCTION

The thrill, excitement, and adventure of moving water draws increasing numbers of canoers and kayakers each year. Moving water has exhilarating challenges for everyone, from the seasoned expert to the novice paddler. Canoeing and kayaking on moving water can be safe and enjoyable when everyone is careful. Unfortunately, emergencies occur. This chapter will help you to recognize, prevent, and respond to canoeing and kayaking emergencies on moving water.

MOVING-WATER SAFETY

Moving water is more powerful than flat water, and presents several types of hazards not found in flat water. Moving-water hazards include long swims in cold water, low-head dams, strainers, hydraulics, entrapment in a craft, and foot entrapment. (See Appendix A for these and other common river hazards.)

To prevent accidents, injuries, and fatalities on moving-water, you need to understand their causes. Most moving-water fatalities can be prevented if paddlers wear their life jackets, avoid the use of alcohol, and protect themselves from the hypothermic effects of cold water.

Guidelines for Moving-Water Safety

In addition to the safe canoeing and kayaking guidelines learned in Chapters 4 and 5, the following additional guidelines should be followed when canoeing and kayaking on moving water:

- Have appropriate paddling skills.
- Know how to read a river and recognize common river hazards (see Appendix A).
- Scout unknown and potentially hazardous water from shore.
- Portage around potential hazards and water beyond your ability.
- Know the different classes of moving water (Appendix B).
- Wear a properly fitted, Coast Guard-approved life jacket that is designed for paddling on moving water.
- If canoeing or kayaking in a decked craft, canoeing with **thigh straps**, or paddling on difficult rapids, wear a helmet.
- Obtain river information through maps and guidebooks before paddling.
- Check water and weather conditions before paddling.

SUPERVISION AND COMMUNICATION ON MOVING WATER

Paddlers, whether in the same or different craft, must be able to communicate with each other. Prior to paddling, review any predetermined hand or whistle signals with all paddlers (for example, one short whistle blast to get someone's attention, or three hard whistle blasts to indicate an emergency).

The American Whitewater Affiliation (AWA) Universal River Signals (Figs. 8-1 to 8-3) are hand and paddle signals used to communicate on moving water, where the sound of the river can make it difficult to hear voices.

Figure 8-1

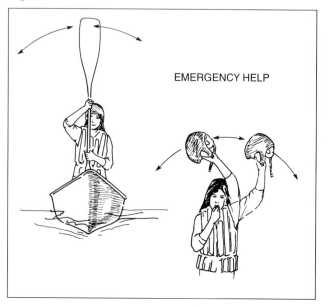

EMERGENCY HELP

Figure 8-2

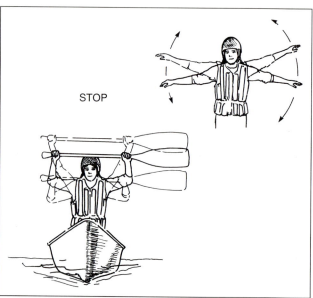

STOP

Source: American Canoeing Association, *Canoeing and Kayaking IM*. Figures 8-1 to 8-3 reprinted with permission.

CHAPTER 8 *Moving-Water Safety—Canoeing and Kayaking*

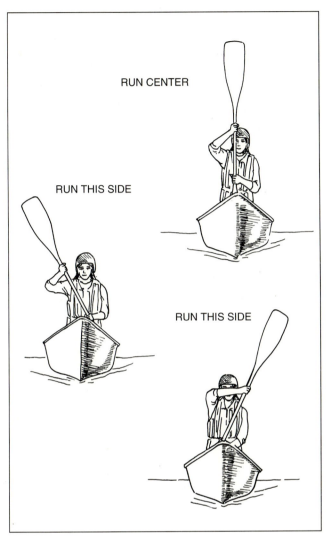

Figure 8-3

When leading a trip or supervising others on moving water, the communication, leader location, and leader-to-participant ratios learned in Chapter 2 may need to be adjusted. Potential moving-water hazards need to be communicated, the leader-to-participant ratio may need to be increased, and the lead, sweep, and other craft may need to give each other more space in order to prevent collisions.

MOVING-WATER EMERGENCIES

Self-Rescue in Moving Water

Capsizes and Falls Overboard
Capsizes, falls overboard, and collisions are common paddling accidents on moving water. Some different rescue techniques are used in moving-water rescue that are not used in flat water.

If your boat capsizes or you fall overboard into moving water—

1. Float downstream on your back with your feet in front of you (Fig. 8-4). This will help you to fend off rocks and avoid entrapping your feet.
2. Swim toward shore or into an *eddy* as soon as it is safe to do so (Fig. 8-5). If you are close to shore, if the water is cold, or if there are hazards further downstream, consider swimming toward shore.
   - In shallow water, swim on your back at an angle against the current and toward shore.
   - In deep water, swim on your front at an angle against the current and toward shore.
3. Do not stand up, you could catch your foot under a rock and become entrapped and pinned, even in just a few feet of water.

The Power of Moving Water

As the speed of water increases, the force of the water on an object increases exponentially. If a current of 3-feet-per-second exerts a force of 17 foot-pounds on your legs, you might reasonably think that a 6-feet-per-second current would exert a force of 34 foot-pounds. This is not so. The force of water increases in proportion to the square of the velocity of the current. If the current velocity doubles, the force of the water increases fourfold.

Current Velocity		Average Total Force of Water (foot-pounds)		
(feet per second)	(miles per hour)	(on legs)	(on body)	(on swamped boat)
3	2	16.8	33.6	168
6	4	67.2	134.0	672
9	6	151.0	302.0	1512
12	8	269.0	538.0	2688

Source: Les Bechdel and Slim Ray, *River Rescue*, with modifications

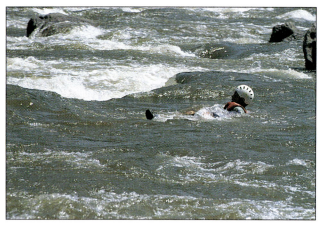

Figure 8-4

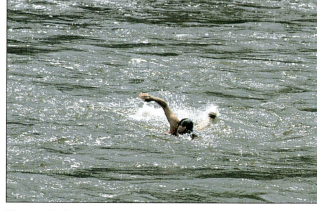

Figure 8-5

4. If necessary or practical, hold on to the craft for flotation (Fig. 8-6).
   - Hold on to the painter or grab loop, keeping the craft in front of you.
   - Stay on the upstream end of the craft to avoid being caught between the craft and a rock.
   - Try to swim with the craft toward shore or into an eddy as soon as possible.
   - If necessary, let go of the craft and swim for shore.
5. Stay alert for assistance from another boat or rescuer.
   - When holding on to a throw bag rope, float on your back so you can breathe.
   - Hold the rope over the shoulder that is furthest from shore, and let the current swing you to shore.

Holes, Hydraulics, and Low-Head Dams

When water flows forcefully down over a rock, ledge, or other obstruction in a river, it forms a depression or *hole*. If the downward flow is strong enough, surface water curls back on itself, forming a strong, recirculating upstream current, called a *hydraulic* (Fig. 8-7). Although small holes or hydraulics may not be particularly dangerous, larger ones with strong recirculating water pose a definite risk.

Low-head dams are barriers built across streams and rivers to control the flow of water (Fig. 8-8). Dangerous hydraulics are formed by low-head dams which can easily trap and hold a person or craft. When approaching a low-head dam from upstream, the waterline may look unusually smooth and calm and may not be visible.

1. To avoid this hazard, stay out of areas with low-head dams or portage around such areas.
2. If you are caught in a low-head dam, do not fight it.
3. Do not panic. Time your breathing with the flow of the hydraulic as it pulls you underwater and recirculates you to the surface and back underwater.
4. If possible, submerge to the bottom, and then swim downstream with the current to reach the surface. Beware, there may be trapped debris circulating in the low-head dam.

Figure 8-6

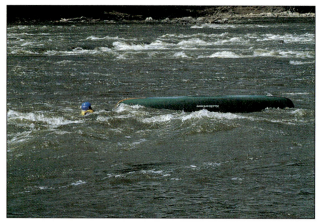

Figure 8-7

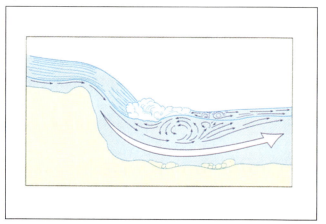

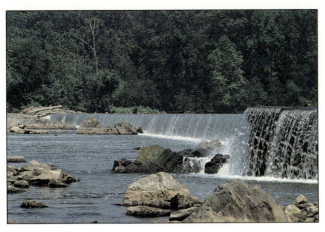

Figure 8-8

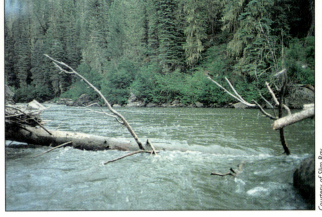

Figure 8-9

Strainers

A *strainer* is an obstacle in a river, often a fallen tree snarled with branches and other debris, that acts like a colander. Water is forced through the obstacle, entrapping or "straining" debris and people (Fig 8-9).

Avoid strainers by paddling or portaging around them. If you fall overboard and are approaching a strainer, avoid entrapment by performing the following steps:

1. Swim toward the strainer head-first with arms extended, ready to grab hold of the object.
2. Kick with your feet behind you at the surface.
3. When you reach the strainer, kick aggressively, keeping your feet at the surface, and climb up onto or over the strainer (Fig. 8-10).

Entrapment in a Canoe or Kayak

The force of the current can trap a person between the craft and a rock or obstacle, or collapse the craft, trapping a paddler inside. This is usually the result of a **broach pin** (Fig. 8-11) or **vertical pin.**

To prevent this dangerous situation:

1. Keep your craft pointed downstream when paddling on moving water.
2. If you collide sideways against a rock, lean downstream toward the rock and try to push the craft off the obstacle with your paddle or hand to keep the craft from filling with water.
3. If your craft starts to fill with water, quickly get out of the boat and onto the rock.
4. Never get between a pinned boat and a rock or other obstacle.

Foot Entrapment

Your feet can become wedged in between or underneath rocks or other submerged objects in fast-moving water (Fig. 8-12). Powerful currents can easily push you underwater and pin you, even in shallow water. To prevent **foot entrapment**—

1. Do not try to stand up in moving water.
2. If you fall overboard, float downstream on your back with your feet in front of you, unless you are approaching a strainer.

Figure 8-10

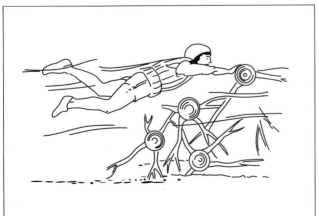

Figure 8-11

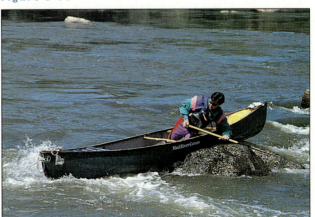

Small Craft Safety

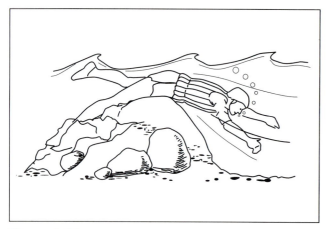

Figure 8-12

Rescuing Others in Moving Water

The methods for assisting others described in Chapter 3 can be safe and effective for rescues in moving water with slight modifications.

Throw Bag Assist with Belay

The throw bag is light, compact, and effective for moving water. As a result, it is one of the most commonly used pieces of rescue equipment for paddlers. The throw bag assist is especially useful in moving-water situations where reaching or wading assists are impractical or unsafe. It can also be used to pendulum a paddler who is stranded on a rock into shore. The throw bag should be used from shore, not from inside a craft. To perform a throw bag assist with belay—

1. Hold the end loop of the line with one hand. Do not put the loop around your wrist.
2. Shout to get the victim's attention. Make eye contact and say that you are going to throw the rope. Tell the victim to grab the rope.
3. With the other hand, throw the bag with an underhand motion (Fig. 8-13, A).
4. Throw the bag as close to the victim as possible so that the line drops within reach.
5. Belay the line for additional holding power.
   - Position the line of the throw bag around the back of your hips (Fig. 8-13, B). Do not tie the rope around any part of your body.
   - Hold on to the tight end of the rope with one hand. With the other hand, hold the loose end of the rope in front of your thighs (Fig. 8-13, C).
   - Brace yourself with a wide stance and let the current swing the victim toward shore (Fig. 8-13, D).
   - Pull the victim to safety using a hand-over-hand motion.

Team Wading Assist

The team wading assist is a wading assist made by a group of two or more people. It can be used to gain access to pinned boats if the water is not too deep and can also be used to reach foot entrapment victims. The advantage of this rescue is that it is simple and can be organized quickly.

The disadvantage of this rescue method is that the rescuers must enter the water. Rescuers risk entrapping their own feet by walking out to the victim. However, the risk of foot entrapment can be minimized by moving in a controlled manner with support. Rescuers also risk being swept downstream in powerful water. This rescue should be used only in shallow, less powerful water.

Follow these steps for a team wading assist:

1. Place a rescuer(s) downstream on the shore with a throw bag in case one of the rescuers or the victim is washed downstream.
2. Have two to five rescuers form a huddle.
3. Rescuers grasp the life jacket of each person beside them at the shoulder (Fig. 8-14).
4. Rescuers move through the river in a controlled manner. One person moves at a time with support from the stationary rescuers.
5. As a team, slowly wade out to the victim.
6. Once you have reached the victim, recover the victim and wade back to shore.[1]

---

[1] Rescue 3 International: *Swiftwater Rescue Technician TM I—with modifications*

Retrieving a Pinned Craft

When canoeing or kayaking on moving water, it is not uncommon for a craft to be pinned against a rock or other obstacle. Follow these guidelines to retrieve a pinned craft in any situation:

- Use the KISS (Keep It Safe & Simple) principle. Since it is a craft and not a person, take your time. Use safe methods, and start with the simplest methods first.
- You may be able to push or pull the craft from the rock it is pinned on. Be careful not to slip between the craft and the rock.
- A line can be attached to the end of the craft, to several points on the craft, or wrapped around the craft, and several people can try to pull it off the object. Try pulling from different angles if you meet resistance. One end of the craft may be more likely to swing free than the other.
- If you are still unable to retrieve the craft, more complicated methods of setting up lines, anchor points, and pulleys can give you a mechanical advantage. These hauling systems require specialized equipment and training.

CHAPTER 8 Moving-Water Safety—Canoeing and Kayaking   75

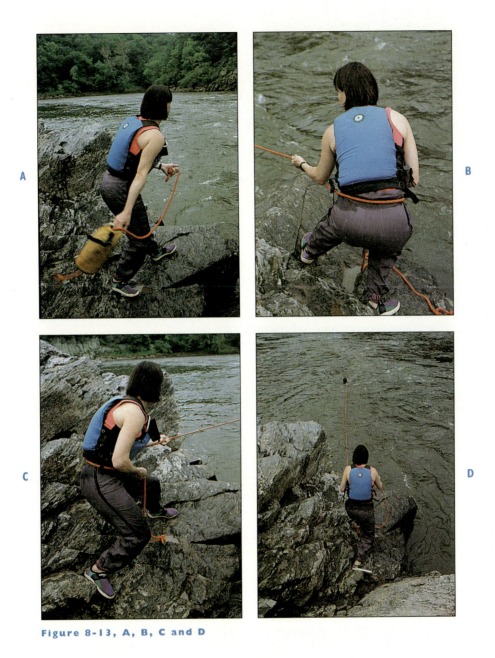

Figure 8-13, A, B, C and D

Figure 8-14

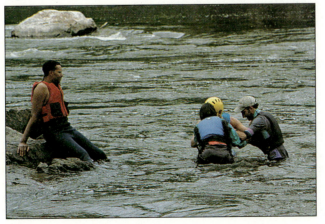

SMALL CRAFT SAFETY

SUMMARY

Canoeing and kayaking on moving water can be safe and enjoyable as well as thrilling and exciting. By recognizing potential hazards in the moving-water environment, and knowing how to prevent moving-water accidents, injuries, and fatalities, you can help provide for a memorable adventure. Effective supervision and communication while paddling on moving water is essential. Having the ability to rescue yourself and assist others in moving water will also help provide for a safe and enjoyable paddling experience.

LEARNING ACTIVITIES

TRUE OR FALSE

1. If you fall into moving water, you should stand up and wade to shore.   True or False?

2. Portage around potential hazards and water beyond your ability to prevent emergencies.   True or False?

3. If you are caught in a low-head dam, swim against the current at an angle.   True or False?

4. When your canoe or kayak is pinned against rocks or other obstructions, you should lean upstream to prevent it from filling with water.   True or False?

5. Most moving-water accidents, injuries, and fatalities can be prevented if paddlers wear their life jackets, avoid the use of alcohol, and protect themselves from the hypothermic affects of cold water.   True or False?

MULTIPLE CHOICE

Circle the letter of the best answer or answers.

1. What are the guidelines for moving-water safety:
   a. Have appropriate paddling skills before going onto moving water.
   b. Know how to read a river, recognize common river hazards, and know the different classes of moving water.
   c. Scout unknown and potentially hazardous water from shore, and portage around potential hazards and water beyond your ability.
   d. Lean upstream if your craft collides sideways against a rock or obstacle.
   e. Wear a properly fitted, Coast Guard-approved life jacket designed for paddling on moving water.

2. Which of the following does *not* help paddlers communicate more effectively on moving water?
   a. Recognizing and understanding the AWA universal river signals for communication among paddlers.
   b. Reviewing hand and whistle signals with all paddlers prior to paddling.
   c. Increasing the lead-to-sweep ratio.
   d. Knowing the whistle signal for a paddling emergency.

3. To help stay safe when paddling moving water, it is best to—
   a. Prevent capsizes, falls overboard, and collisions.
   b. Practice swimming through strainers and low-head dams.
   c. Recognize and avoid moving-water hazards.
   d. Scout potentially hazardous water after paddling it.

4. If you capsize or fall overboard in a canoe or kayak, what should you do to rescue yourself?
   a. Float downstream on your back with your feet in front of you.
   b. Swim toward shore or into an eddy as soon as it is safe to do so.
   c. Do not stand up.
   d. If necessary or practical, hold onto the craft for protection.
   e. Be alert for assistance from another boat or rescuer.
   f. All of the above.

5. If your craft collides sideways against a rock or object, you should—
   a. Lean downstream toward the rock to keep the craft from filling with water.
   b. Try to push the craft off the obstacle with your paddle or hand if it fills with water.
   c. Try to get between the craft and the rock to unpin it.
   d. a and b.

CHAPTER 8 *Moving-Water Safety—Canoeing and Kayaking*

FILL IN

Fill in the correct answers.

1. Moving-water hazards include hydraulics and entrapment in a broached craft. List at least two other hazards for canoers or kayakers on moving water.
   _____
   _____

2. List at least three guidelines for moving-water safety.
   _____
   _____
   _____
   _____
   _____

3. List the missing steps for self-rescue if your boat capsizes or you fall overboard.
   1. _____
   2. Swim toward shore or into an eddy as soon as it is safe to do so.
   3. _____
   4. If necessary or practical, hold onto the craft for flotation.
   5. _____

4. Fill in the missing moving-water hazard for each of the following.
   a. Swim toward the _____ head-first with arms extended, ready to grab hold of the object.
   b. If you are caught in a(n) _____, do not fight it.
   c. If your craft is pinned against a rock or obstacle, lean against the downstream side to avoid a(n) _____.
   d. To prevent a(n) _____ do not try to stand up in moving water.

5. The throw bag assist with belay is especially useful for rescuing a capsized paddler in what moving-water situations? _____
   _____

SCENARIO

1. You are responsible for leading a group of young novice paddlers down a stretch of river with class I and II rapids. You have canoed the river before, but most of the paddlers have only been on flat water. During the trip, one of the canoes hits a rock sideways about thirty feet from shore. Not knowing what to do, the paddlers lean upstream away from the rock. The canoe flips over and fills with water. One of the paddlers manages to climb onto the rock, but the other is in the water heading downstream.

   a. Who is in the most danger, the paddler on the rock, the broached canoe, or the paddler in the water?
   _____

   b. What could the paddler in the water do for self-rescue? _____
   _____

   c. What could you do to assist the paddler in the water? _____
   _____

   d. How could you safely assist the paddler on the rock? _____
   _____

See answers to learning activities on page 85.

Glossary

Active drowning victim: A person exhibiting universal behavior that includes struggling at the surface for 20 to 60 seconds before submerging.
Air bags: Flotation materials placed inside a kayak to provide buoyancy for the craft.
Beach drag: A method of pulling an unconscious or heavy victim out of the water on a sloping shore or beach by gripping the victim under the armpits and walking backward toward shore.
Beam: The width of a craft at its widest point.
Belay: To anchor a line by positioning it around the back of your hips.
Broach pin: When a craft is pushed sideways against a rock or obstacle, and held there by the force of the current.
Boom: A wooden or metal pole attached to the mast that holds out the bottom of a sail.
Bow: The front of the craft.
Canoe: A light, slender boat with a pointed bow and pointed or square stern, generally propelled by single-blade paddles.
Capalene: An insulated material used in making winter clothing.
Capsize: To turn a craft upside down in the water.
Centerboard: An inserted or pivoting plate of wood, fiberglass, or metal that projects below the bottom of a sailboat to help prevent the boat from sliding sideways due to the wind; some types of centerboards are also called daggerboards.
Coaming: A raised rim around the cockpit to which the spray skirt attaches.
Cockpit: An opening in the kayak where the paddler sits.
Collision: A craft crashing into another craft or object.
Critical Incident Stress: The stress a person experiences during or after a highly stressful emergency.
Deck: The flat surface over the hull that encloses an interior space.
Delayed-help environment: Environment or situation in which help from the emergency medical services (EMS) system would take 30 minutes or more.
Distressed swimmer: A person capable of staying afloat but likely to need assistance to get to safety.

Drowning: Death by suffocation underwater.
Eddy: The sheltered area behind or downstream of an obstruction, where the currents flow upstream toward the obstruction.
Emergency Action Plan (EAP): A written plan detailing how members of a group are to respond in a specific type of emergency.
Emergency Medical Services (EMS) personnel: Trained and equipped community-based personnel dispatched through an emergency number, usually 9-1-1, to provide medical care to victims of injury or sudden illness.
Emergency Medical Services (EMS): Community resources and medical personnel that provide emergency care to victims of injury or sudden illness.
Entrapment in a canoe or kayak: When the force of the current traps a person between the craft and a rock or obstacle, or collapses the boat and traps a paddler inside the craft.
Fall overboard: To unintentionally fall out of a craft into the water.
Float plan: A written plan with details of a boating trip, left with someone ashore.
Flat water: Lake water or river current where no rapids exist and eddies are slight.
Foot entrapment: When a person's foot is wedged between or underneath rocks or another submerged object in moving water.
Grab loop: A coil of line connected to the stern or bow of the kayak used to grab the craft.
Gunwale (pronounced "gunnel"): The top edge of the sides of a craft.
Head splint: A technique used to stabilize the head, neck, and back of a person with a suspected spinal injury.
Heaving line: A floating rope of a highly visible color used for water rescue.
Heaving jug: A homemade piece of rescue equipment for throwing to a victim, made of a 1-gallon plastic container containing about half an inch of water, with 50 to 75 feet of floating line attached.

Glossary

Heel: When a boat leans over to one side because of the pressure of wind on the sail(s).
HELP position: A position for floating in cold water while awaiting rescue in which you draw up your knees, hold your arms at your sides, and fold your lower arms against your chest. (HELP = Heat Escape Lessening Posture.)
Hip and shoulder support: A technique used to stabilize the head, neck, and back of a victim with a suspected spinal injury.
Hole: A type of hydraulic that is formed by a rock, ledge, or other obstruction in a river.
Huddle position: A position for two or more people floating in cold water while awaiting rescue, in which you put your arms over each other's shoulders so that the sides of your chests are together; children and/or elderly persons are placed in the middle of the huddle.
Hull: The main body of a craft.
Hydraulic: Strong force created by water flowing downward over an obstruction and then reversing its flow.
Hypothermia: A life-threatening condition in which the body is unable to maintain warmth and the entire body cools.
Incident report: A report filed by the group leader or assistant(s) involved in any way in a rescue or other emergency.
Jibe: To change from one tack to another when sailing downwind.
Kapok: A fiber used in to fill life jackets and other flotation devices.
Kayak: A decked boat with pointed ends and a cockpit, propelled by a double-blade paddle.
Keel: The weighted underwater fin on the hull, which helps provide stability and prevents the boat from slipping sideways. *Also*, The centerline of a boat running from the bow to the stern.
Lawsuit: A legal procedure for settling a dispute.
Lead craft: The front or first craft in a group of craft.
Leeward: In the opposite direction from the wind source, or downwind.
Liability: A legal responsibility.
Life jacket: A type of personal flotation device (PFD) that can be worn.
Low-head dam: A barrier built across streams and rivers to control the flow of water.
Main sheet: The line used to pull in or let out the mainsail.
Mainsail: The sail attached to the mast and boom.
Mast: The vertical wooden or metal pole in a sailboat that holds up the sail.
Murky: Dark or cloudy.
Negligence: The failure to provide the level of care a person of similar training would be expected to provide, thereby causing injury or damage to another.

Oars: The bladed devices used to move a rowboat through the water.
Open water: Natural bodies of water, such as lakes, ponds, rivers, streams, and the ocean.
Outfit: To furnish a canoe with safety equipment, provisions, and gear.
Painter: A line attached to the bow and/or stern of the craft.
Passive drowning victim: An unconscious victim facedown, submerged, or near the surface of the water.
Personal Flotation Device (PFD): Life jacket, buoyancy vest, wearable flotation aid, throwable flotation aid, deck suit, work vest, sailboarding vest, or hybrid inflatable flotation aid.
Polypropylene: A light, highly water-resistant thermoplastic material.
Port: The left side of a craft.
Portage: To carry a boat and supplies from one body of water to another, or around an obstacle.
Reaching assist: A method of helping someone out of the water by reaching to that person with an object.
Rescue breathing: A technique of breathing for a non-breathing victim.
Rescue tube: A vinyl, foam-filled, floating support used in rescuing someone in the water.
Rigging: The lines and fittings used to adjust the sails.
Ring buoy: A rescue device made of buoyant cork, kapok, or other plastic-covered material with an attached line, for throwing to a victim in the water.
Rocker: The curve of the keel from bow to stern. The greater the curve, the less resistance to turning.
Rowboat: A small, open boat propelled by oars.
Rudder: A flat projection in the water used to steer the boat.
Rules of the Road: Navigation rules indicating right-of-way among boats to prevent collisions.
Sailboat: A boat with one or more sails, powered by wind.
Safety boat: A boat used for supervising or recovering other craft, also known as a chase boat.
Safety position: When a boat is stopped with its sails eased and flapping, and the wind coming from the side.
Seizure: A disorder in the brain's electrical activity, marked by loss of consciousness and often uncontrollable muscle movement.
Shepherd's crook: A long pole with a hook on the end that can be used to pull a conscious drowning victim to safety.
Spray skirt: Material worn around a paddler's waist and attached to the coaming. It prevents water from entering the kayak.

Glossary

Standard of care: The degree of care expected from a reasonable and careful person under the same or similar circumstances.
Starboard: The right side of a craft.
Stern: The back of a craft.
Stern seat: The back seat of a craft.
Survival floating: A face-down floating technique used in warm water while awaiting rescue.
Strainer: An obstacle in a river, often a fallen tree snarled with branches and other debris, that acts like a colander. Water is forced through the obstacle, entrapping or "straining" debris and people.
Swamp: To fill with water.
Sweep craft: The craft that brings up the rear to ensure that no one is left behind.
Tack: The orientation of a boat based on the side of the boat nearer the wind (i.e., a starboard tack or port tack). Also, to change from one tack to another when sailing upwind.
Tandem: Two people paddling together in a canoe or small craft.
Thigh straps: Straps which hold you firmly in a canoe for stability on rough water.

Throw bag: A nylon bag containing 50 to 75 feet of coiled floating line used in water rescue.
Throwing assist: A method of helping someone out of the water by throwing a floating object with a line attached.
Thwarts (stern, center, and bow): Support braces in a canoe which go from gunwale to gunwale.
Tiller: The handle attached to the top of a rudder used to steer the craft.
Transom: The flat vertical back end of a rowboat.
Trim: The balance of a craft from front to back.
Vertical pin: When a craft becomes pinned vertically against a rock or obstacle.
Walking assist: A method to help a person walk out from shallow water with the rescuer holding on to the person.
Waves: A ridge or swell moving along the surface of a body of water.
Wet exit: A self-rescue method of exiting a capsized kayak.
Windward: In the direction toward the wind source, or upwind.

Learning Activity Answers

Chapter 1

True or False
1. F 2. F 3. T 4. T 5. T 6. F 7. T

Multiple Choice
1. e 2. a, c, d 3. a, c, d, e 4. b, c, e 5. c 6. d

Fill In
1. Four people (4 2/3, rounded down)
2. Murky water, weeds, tides, currents, flooding, fast-moving water, cold water, hidden rocks, debris, low-head dams, hydraulics, steep drops, dams, falls, strainers, hazardous obstacles, waves, sandbars

Scenario
1a. Learn about swimming, boating, CPR, and first aid; contact your local Red Cross for information about swimming, CPR, and first aid courses; check with your local Red Cross, the U.S. Coast Guard, state boating officials, and other organizations about boating courses (see appendix C for a list of boating and other water safety organizations); always supervise children in, on, or around the water; know how to respond to a small craft emergency; do not attempt a swimming rescue unless you have specialized training and proper equipment; you can help a victim only if you stay safe yourself; wear a U.S. Coast Guard–approved life jacket when boating; be aware of potential water hazards; pay attention to local weather conditions and forecasts; know how to prevent accidents, recognize hazards, and care for injuries.
1b. Murky water, weeds, hidden rocks, debris, obstructions, and currents
1c. Do not lean over or sit on the gunwale; keep your weight centered in the craft; when moving around in a boat, have two hands and one foot, or one hand and two feet in contact with the boat; look out for other craft and submerged objects; follow the rules of the road.
1d. Yes
1e. 80 percent of boaters who drown are not wearing a life jacket; a life jacket will keep you afloat, help conserve body heat, and can protect you from the impact of rocks, debris, or another craft, but only if you *have it on;* boating accidents happen quickly and unexpectedly, and you will not have time to put your life jacket on, or may not even be able to find it.

Chapter 2

True or False
1. F 2. T 3. F 4. T 5. F

Multiple Choice
1. e 2. e 3. a 4. d 5. c

Fill In
1. Growing cloud cover and darkening skies, sudden changes in wind velocity or direction, gusty winds, lightning, thunder, increasing waves, sudden temperature changes
2. float plan
3. Life jackets for each person, a type IV (throwable) PFD, throw bag, extra line/rope, extra paddles/oars, bailers and sponges, first aid kit in a waterproof container, flares, blankets, a means of communication—such as a cellular phone or two-way radio, a sound device—such as an air horn or whistle, a visual distress signal—such as a flare, strobe light, signal mirror, chemical light stick, or colored dye marker

Scenario
a. 1. Be aware of the conditions and potential hazards of the water environment, whether it is a pool, lake, river, ocean, or other body of water. Know its unique conditions as well as hazards common in your geographical area, such as storms.
2. Understand the various recreational activities that are common in the water environment. Consider the age and ability of participants in those activities.
3. Learn what kind of accidents and injuries have occurred in the past in the water environment. This will help you prevent further injuries and be prepared for aquatic emergencies.
4. Have the appropriate safety equipment and supplies for your water environment (see page 14).

Learning Activity Answers 83

b. Life jackets for each person on board ; a type IV (throwable) PFD; throw bag; extra line/rope; extra paddles/oars; bailers and sponges; blankets; a sound device, such as an air horn or whistle
c. Selecting a leader; knowing the responsibilities and legal considerations; selecting the locale and route; checking the weather conditions; checking the water conditions; choosing the appropriate clothing; selecting and checking the appropriate equipment; preparing for possible emergencies
d. Consider their limits, skill level, and experience; be aware of and responsive to medical conditions or restrictions that participants may have; ask participants to communicate their abilities, limitations, or other considerations to you.

Chapter 3

True or False
1. F   2. F   3. T   4. F   5. F

Multiple Choice
1. a   2. e   3. c   4. c   5. b, c, d

Fill In
1. reaching; throwing
2. A person having a seizure can lose consciousness and slip under the water without warning. Also, he or she may inhale water into the lungs, leading to a life-threatening condition.
3. A fall from a height greater than the person's height; any person found unconsciousness for an unknown reason; any serious head injury; any injury from using a diving board or water slide, or from diving from a height, such as a bank or a cliff; diving into shallow water
4. hip and shoulder support; head splint.
5. HELP position—draw your knees up to your chest; keep your face forward and out of the water; hold your upper arms at your sides; and fold your lower arms against or across your chest.
   Huddle position—with two people, put your arms over each other so sides of chests are together; with three or more people, put your arms over each other's shoulders so that the sides of your chests are together; place children or elderly persons in the middle of the huddle.

Scenarios
1. a. 4
   b. Pole; shepherd's crook; oar; paddle; tree branch; shirt; belt; towel
   c. 1. Brace yourself in the craft, on the pier surface or on the shoreline.
      2. Extend the object to the victim.
      3. When the victim grasps the object, slowly and carefully pull him to safety, keep your body low and lean back to avoid being pulled into the water.
   d. throwing assist
   e. Ring buoy; buoyant cushion; heaving line; throw bag; rescue tube; picnic jug; or extra life jacket
   f. 1. Get into a stride position: the leg opposite your throwing arm is forward. This helps to keep your balance when you throw the object.
      2. Step on the end of the line with your forward foot.
      3. Shout to get the victim's attention; make eye contact and say that your are going to throw the object now; tell the victim to grab it.
      4. Bend your knees and throw the object to the victim; try to throw the object upwind and/or up current, just over the victim's head, so the line drops within reach.
      5. When the victim has grasped the object or the line, slowly pull him or her to safety.
      6. If the object does not reach the victim, quickly pull the line back in and throw it again; try to keep the line from tangling but do not waste time trying to recoil it; if the object is a throw bag, partially fill the bag with some water and throw it again.
2. a. Have someone call 9-1-1 or the local emergency number.
   b. Support the child to keep the child's head and face above water.
   c. Take the child out of the water, and place the child on his or her side to let fluids drain from the mouth; provide emergency care if needed.

Chapter 4

Page 39 Learning Activity Answers
1. Gunwale   2. Bow   3. Hull   4. Thwarts   5. Stern
6. Painter

True or False
1. F   2. F   3. T

Multiple Choice
1. d   2. c   3. a, b, d

Fill In
1. thwarts
2. Keep your weight low by paddling in a kneeling position; when moving around in a canoe, have two hands and one foot or one hand and two feet in contact with the craft; passengers should sit on the bottom of the canoe; watch out for submerged objects, potential hazards, and other boats.
3. 1. People   2. Craft and gear
4. To stabilize it.

Scenarios
1. a. Yes
   b. Standing up
   c. Yes
   d. 1. From the side of the canoe hold onto the gunwale with one hand and a thwart with the other hand.

2. Keeping your weight on the gunwale and thwart, kick vigorously to raise your hips to the gunwale.
3. Rotate your hips to sit inside the canoe, then bring your legs into the craft.
4. Carefully maintain your balance, and steady the craft while your partner enters the canoe.

2. 1. Roll the canoe over so the bottom is up and position it perpendicular to your craft.
   2. Lift one end of the upside-down canoe onto the gunwale, near the middle of your canoe. At the same time, have one of the paddlers in the water push down on the end of the canoe that is in the water.
   3. Carefully slide the upside-down canoe across the gunwales of your craft.
   4. Roll the canoe upright while still across the gunwales, and then slide it back into the water.
   5. The paddlers can then reenter their canoe as you hold the two canoes side-by-side for stability.

Chapter 5

Page 47 Learning Activity Answers
1. Bow   2. Grab loops   3. Deck   4. Cockpit
5. Coaming   6. Stern   7. Air bag

True or False
1. F   2. T   3. F   4. F

Multiple Choice
1. c   2. b   3. e   4. a, c, d, e

Fill In
1. slowly and deliberately
2. helmet
3. 1. People
   2. The kayak (if it does not put you in danger); gear (if it does not put you in danger)
4. Have the victim hold onto the stern of your kayak while you tow him or her to shore.

Scenarios
1. a. A wet exit (exit the kayak)
   b. 1. Release the spray skirt from the coaming.
      2. Push yourself out of the kayak with both hands on the sides of the craft.
      3. Tuck your body forward and pull your legs out together.
      4. Surface, hold onto the grab loop, and swim with it to shore.
2. 1. Have the capsized paddler hold onto the stern of your craft.
   2. From your craft, turn the kayak upside down in the water.
   3. Pull the upside-down kayak up onto your deck.
   4. Balance the upside-down kayak across your deck, and rock it from one end to the other to empty the water out of the cockpit.
   5. Lean your craft from side to side to assist the rocking motion. If necessary, have the capsized paddler assist rocking the kayak by pulling down the high end of the kayak.
   6. Once the kayak is empty of water, roll it upright and slide it back into the water.
   7. Assist the person into their kayak by bracing it alongside yours with the paddles across both craft and have the person climb on board as you stabilize the craft.

Chapter 6

Page 54 Learning Activity Answers
1. Starboard   2. Rudder   3. Tiller   4. Mast   5. Port
6. Main sheet   7. Stern   8. Hull   9. Boom   10. Bow
11. Gunwale   12. Centerboard

True or False
1. T   2. F   3. T   4. T

Multiple Choice
1. a;   2. c;   3. b;   4. a, b, c

Fill In
1. Wear your life jacket; prevent collisions; prevent capsizing; prevent falling overboard
2. carelessness; ignorance of the rules of the road
3. stay with the boat
4. 1. People   2. Craft and gear
5. A sudden gust of wind can catch a sailor by surprise and overpower the boat; a poorly executed jibe can unbalance the boat and make it suddenly heel or tip to one side; a broken tiller can cause the operator to lose control; letting go of the tiller or main sheet can cause a sudden change in the angle of heel; a quick turn in heavy winds can cause the boat to roll over.

Scenarios
1. a. Stay with the boat.
   b. 1. Rotate the boat so the bow faces the wind.
      2. While holding onto the gunwale and the centerboard, swing the boat upright. If more weight is needed, carefully stand on the centerboard, hold onto the gunwale, and swing the sailboat upright.
      3. Reboard the boat at the stern.
   c. Hold onto the boat or climb up onto the hull and signal for help.
   d. You will be safer and rescuers can see you better.
2. 1. Alert other crew members on board by shouting "crew overboard." Keep the victim in sight and tack as soon as possible.

2. Approach from downwind. This minimizes the danger of hitting the victim with the sailboat as you approach.
3. Place your sailboat in the safety position next to the victim.
4. Have the victim enter at the stern of the sailboat. If the victim needs assistance, reach with a life jacket or other object and pull him or her to the stern of the sailboat. If the victim cannot hold onto the life jacket, grasp the victim, pull him or her to the stern, and help the person on board.

Chapter 7

Page 63 Learning Activity Answers
1. Hull 2. Stern 3. Stern seat 4. Bow 5. Transom
6. Gunwale

True or False
1. T 2. T 3. F 4. F

Multiple Choice
1. c 2. c 3. a, b, c, e 4. d 5. a

Fill In
1. Wear a life jacket; know how to prevent capsizes; know how to prevent falls overboard
2. stay with the boat
3. Ring buoy; throw bag; rescue tube; heaving line; buoyant cushion; life jacket; homemade device
4. 1. People
   2. Craft and gear
5. be safer with the boat; will be able to see you better

Scenarios
1. a. 1. Place your hands on the transom.
      2. Kick vigorously, and raise your hips while keeping your weight on the transom.
      3. Rotate your hips and sit on the stern seat, or in the back of the craft.
      4. Swing your legs into the rowboat.
   b. Stay with the boat and signal for help.
2. a. Reaching assist
   b. 1. Approach the person with the stern end of the boat.
      2. From the stern, reach an oar, extra life jacket, or other object to the person.
      3. Pull the person to the stern.
      4. Assist the person over the transom into the stern of the craft.

Chapter 8

True or False
1. F 2. T 3. F 4. F 5. T

Multiple Choice
1. a, b, c, e 2. c 3. a, c 4. f 5. a

Fill In
1. Long swims in cold water, low-head dams, strainers, and foot entrapments
2. Have appropriate paddling skills; know how to read a river and recognize common river hazards; scout unknown and potentially hazardous water from shore; portage around potential hazards and water beyond your ability; know the different classes of moving water; wear a properly fitted, Coast Guard-approved life jacket that is designed for paddling on moving water; obtain information on the river through maps and guidebooks before canoeing; check water and weather conditions before paddling.
3. a. Float downstream on your back with your feet in front of you.
   c. Do not stand up, you could catch your foot under a rock and become entrapped and pinned, even in just a few feet of water.
   e. Be alert for assistance from another boat or rescuer.
4. a. strainer
   b. low-head dam/hydraulic
   c. entrapment in a canoe or kayak
   d. foot entrapment
5. Where reaching or wading assists are impractical or unsafe

Scenario
a. the paddler in the water
b. Swim aggressively to the safest shore, be ready to catch a throw bag.
c. Use a throw bag assist with belay from shore.
d. Use a throw bag assist with belay or team wading assist.

Appendix A: River Hazards

HAZARD	CHARACTERISTICS	PROBLEMS
Gravel Bars	Often not visible and difficult to detect in advance. Frequently cause a river to split into two or more channels.	Can cause a paddler to run into an obstruction in the river. In shallow areas, a paddler may get stuck on a gravel bar.
Chutes and Waves	Chutes are breaks in ledges which can result in fast-moving water. Waves occur at the base of a chute when the fast water meets slower water.	Risk of swamping if the waves are large at the base of the chute.
Pillow	Water that flows over and around a rock. Looks like a pillow on the upstream side of the obstruction.	Can create a hydraulic behind the obstruction. Can cause pinning or a drop on the downriver side.
Hydraulic/Hole	Strong force created by water flowing downward over a rock, ledge, low-head dam, or other obstruction then reversing its flow.	A large hydraulic may swamp or hold a boat and people. Powerful hydraulics are life threatening.

APPENDIX A *River Hazards*

HAZARD	CHARACTERISTICS	PROBLEMS
Vs	*Upstream V* is formed with a rock at the upstream point and a wake, turbulence, or eddy line fanning out from it downstream. *Downstream V* is the result of the intersection of two upstream Vs. It indicates a clear channel between obstructions.	Avoid the point of an upstream V because it indicates a rock or obstruction. Clear channel
Strainer	An obstacle in a river, often a fallen tree snarled with branches and other debris, that acts like a colander, forcing water through the obstacle, entrapping or "straining" debris and people in the river.	Potential entrapment or pinning
Waterfall	Water flowing over steep rocks. Powerful and turbulent water is found downstream and beneath the waterfall. An indicator of a waterfall is a horizon line (straight line across the river)—an area of smooth, calm-looking water followed by a line, indicating that the river drops out of sight and reappears further downstream. Another indication may be the sound of falling water.	Serious injury or death can result.
Low-Head Dam	A barrier built across streams and rivers to control the flow of water. Dangerous hydraulics are formed by low-head dams. An indicator of a dam is a horizon line or the sound of falling water.	A low-head dam, with only a slight vertical drop, can create a hydraulic, which can be virtually impossible to escape from without assistance.

Photo of strainer courtesy of Slim Ray. Photo of low-head dam courtesy of Canadian Red Cross.

Appendix B: The International Scale of River Difficulty

The various combinations of river features give a stream its character and determine its difficulty for paddling. Commonly paddled rivers and streams have been categorized under the International Scale of River Difficulty. This scale has evolved over a period of years and is accepted and utilized by virtually all paddling organizations and river guidebooks. Not only are individual rapids classified in the scale, but an entire section of a river may be so classified.

White Water Classifications

Class I: Easy
Fast moving water with riffles and small waves. Few obstructions, all obvious and easily missed with little training. Risk to swimmers is slight; self-rescue is easy.

Class II: Novice
Straightforward rapids with wide, clear channels which are evident without scouting. Occasional maneuvering may be required, but rocks and medium sized waves are easily missed by trained paddlers. Swimmers are seldom injured and group assistance, while helpful, is seldom needed.

Class III: Intermediate
Rapids with moderate, irregular waves which may be difficult to avoid and which can swamp an open canoe. Complex maneuvers in fast current and good boat control in tight waves or strainers may be present but are easily avoided. Strong eddies and powerful current effects can be found, particularly on large-volume rivers. Scouting is advisable for inexperienced parties. Injuries while swimming are rare; self-rescue is usually easy but group assistance may be required to avoid long swims.

Class IV: Advanced
Intense, powerful but predictable rapids requiring precise boat handling in turbulent water. Depending on the character of the river, it may feature large, unavoidable waves and holes or constricted passages demanding fast maneuvers under pressure. A fast, reliable eddy turn may be needed to initiate maneuvers, scout rapids, or rest. Rapids may require "must" moves about dangerous hazards. Scouting is necessary the first time down. Risk of injury to swimmers is only moderate to high, and water conditions may make self-rescue difficult. Group assistance for rescue is often essential but requires practiced skills. A strong eskimo roll is highly recommended.

Class V: Expert
Extremely long, obstructed, or very violent rapids which expose a paddler to above average endangerment. Drops may contain large, unavoidable waves and holes or steep, congested chutes with complex, demanding routes. Rapids may continue for long distances between pools, demanding a high level of fitness. What eddies exist may be small, turbulent, or difficult to reach. At the high end of the scale, several of these factors may be combined. Scouting is mandatory but often difficult. Swims are dangerous, and rescue is difficult even for experts. A very reliable eskimo roll, proper equipment, extensive experience, and practiced rescue skills are essential for survival.

Class VI: Extreme
One grade more difficult than Class V. These runs often exemplify the extremes of difficulty, unpredictability, and danger. The consequences of errors are very severe and rescue may be impossible. For teams of experts only, at favorable water levels, after close personal inspections and taking all precautions. This does not represent drops thought to be unrunnable, but may include rapids which are only occasionally run.

Source: The American Whitewater Affiliation

**the river should be considered one class more difficult than normal if the water temperature is below 50 degrees F, or if it is an extended trip in a wilderness area.

Appendix C: Small Craft/Water Safety Organizations and Resources

AAHPERD—American Alliance for Health, Physical Education, Recreation and Dance
1900 Association Drive
Reston, VA 22091
(703)476-3400

American Camping Association
5000 State Road 67 N
Martinsville, IN 46151-7902
(317)342-8456

American Canoe Association
7432 Alban Station Blvd. Suite B-226
Springfield, VA 22150
(703)451-0141

American National Red Cross
Health and Safety Services
8111 Gatehouse Road
Falls Church, VA 22042
(703)206-7180

American Sailing Association
13922 Marquesas Way
Marina Del Ray, CA 90292-6000
(310)822-7171

American Whitewater Affiliation
P.O. Box 636
Margaretville, NY 12455
(914)586-2355

Boat/U.S. Foundation
880 S. Pickett Street
Alexandria, VA 22304
(703)823-9550

Boy Scouts of America
1325 West Walnut Hill Lane
Irving, TX 75038
(972)580-2423

Canadian Power and Sail Squadrons
26 Golden Gate Court
Scarborough, Ontario, Canada M1P3A5
(416)293-2438

Canadian Red Cross
1800 Alta Vista Drive
Ottawa, Ontario, Canada K1G4J5
(613)739-2215

Canyonlands Field Institute
Box 68
Moab, UT 84532
(801)259-7750

The Commodore Longfellow Society
2531 Stonington Road
Atlanta, GA 30338

Girl Scouts of the U.S.A.
420 Fifth Avenue
New York, NY 10018
(212)852-8000

National Association of State Boating Law Administrators
2200 N. 33rd Street
Lincoln, NE 68503-0370
(402)471-4479

Nantahala Outdoor Center Programs Office
13077 Highway 19 West
Bryson City, NC 28713-9114
(888)662-1662

National Boating Federation
3217 Fiji Lane
Alameda, CA 94502
(510)523-2098

89

APPENDIX C *Small Craft/Water Safety Organizations and Resources*

National Recreation and Park Association (NRPA)
  Aquatic Section
650 West Higgins Road
Hoffman Estates, IL 60195
(708)843-7529

National Safe Boating Council, Inc.
Administrative Office
P.O. Box 8510
Lexington, KY 40533-8510
(502)867-2037

Professional Paddlesports Association
P.O. Box 248
U.S. 27 & Hornbeck Roads
Butler, KY 41006-9674
(606)472-2205

Rescue III International
P.O. Box 519
Elk Grove, CA 95759-0519
(800)457-3728

U.S. Coast Guard
2100 Second Street, SW, G-OPB-2
Washington, DC 20593-0001
(202)267-1060

U.S. Coast Guard Auxiliary
9449 Watson Industrial Park
St. Louis, MO 63126
(314)962-8828

U.S. Power Squadron
2202 Colonial Drive
League City, TX 77573
(281)334-0559

U.S. Rowing Association
Pan American Plaza, Suite 400
201 South Capitol Ave.
Indianapolis, IN 46225
(317)237-5656

U.S. Canoe and Kayak Team
Pan American Plaza, Suite 610
201 South Capitol Ave
Indianapolis, IN 46225
(317)237-5690

United States Lifesaving Association (USLA)
425 East McFetridge Drive
Chicago, IL 60605
(312)294-2332

United States Sailing Association
P.O. Box 1260
15 Maritime Drive
Portsmouth, RI 02871-6015
(401)683-0800

Wilderness Medical Society
P.O. Box 2463
Indianapolis, IN 46206
(317)631-1745

YMCA of the U.S.A.
101 North Wacker Drive
Chicago, IL 60606
(800)872-9622

YWCA of the U.S.A.
726 Broadway
New York, NY 10003
(212)614-2700

Appendix D*

FLOAT PLAN

Complete this plan, before going boating and leave it with a reliable person who can be depended upon to notify the Coast Guard, or other rescue organization, should you not return as scheduled. Do not file this plan with the Coast Guard.

TODAY'S DATE _____ (if overnight, date returning) _____

1. NAME OF PERSON REPORTING _____
TELEPHONE NUMBER _____

2. DESCRIPTION OF BOAT. TYPE _____
COLOR _____ TRIM _____
REGISTRATION NO. _____ LENGTH _____
NAME _____ MAKE _____
OTHER INFO. _____

3. NUMBER OF PERSONS ABOARD _____
NAME _____ NAME _____
AGE _____ AGE _____
ADDRESS _____ ADDRESS _____
_____ _____
PHONE # _____ PHONE # _____
Please list additional passengers and information on the back of this form.

4. TRIP EXPECTATIONS: LEAVE AT _____ (TIME)
FROM _____
GOING TO _____
EXPECT TO RETURN BY _____ (TIME)
AND IN NO EVENT LATER THAN _____ (TIME)

5. IF NOT RETURNED BY _____ (TIME) CALL THE COAST GUARD, OR
_____ (LOCAL AUTHORITY)
TELEPHONE NUMBERS _____

6. ENGINE TYPE _____ H.P. _____
NO. OF ENGINES _____ FUEL CAPACITY _____

7. SURVIVAL EQUIPMENT: (CHECK AS APPROPRIATE)
☐ PFDs   ☐ FLARES   ☐ MIRROR   ☐ SMOKE SIGNALS
☐ CLOTHING   ☐ FLASHLIGHT   ☐ FOOD   ☐ PADDLES
☐ WATER   ☐ OTHERS   ☐ ANCHOR   ☐ RAFT OR DINGHY
☐ EPIRB

8. RADIO: ☐ YES ☐ NO
TYPE _____ FREQS. _____

9. ANY OTHER PERTINENT INFO. _____
_____

10. AUTOMOBILE LICENSE _____ TYPE _____
TRAILER LICENSE _____ COLOR AND MAKE OF AUTO _____
WHERE PARKED _____

MAKE ADDITIONAL COPIES OF THIS FORM FOR YOUR USE

*Source: USCG Auxiliary, *Boating Safely Instructor's Manual*, 1997.

Appendix E*

ACCIDENT REPORT FORM

DEPARTMENT OF TRANSPORTATION U.S. COAST GUARD CG-3865(REV. X/94)	**BOATING ACCIDENT REPORT**	
	State Assigned Case No. _____	FORM APPROVED OMB NO. 2115-0010

The operator/owner of a vessel used for recreational purposes is required to file a report in writing whenever an accident results in: loss of life or disappearance from a vessel; an injury that requires medical treatment beyond first aid; or property damage in excess of $500 or complete loss of the vessel. Reports in death and injury cases must be submitted within 48 hours. Reports in other cases must be submitted within 10 days. Reports must be submitted to the reporting authority in the state where the accident occurred. This form is provided to assist the operator in filing the required written report.

COMPLETE ALL BLOCKS (indicate those not applicable by "N/A")

ACCIDENT DATA

DATE OF ACCIDENT	TIME am pm	NAME OF BODY OF WATER	LOCATION (Give location precisely)	
NUMBER OF VESSELS INVOLVED	NEAREST CITY OR TOWN	COUNTY	STATE	ZIP CODE

WEATHER (check all that apply)	WATER CONDITIONS	TEMPERATURE (estimate)	WIND	VISIBILITY
[ ] Clear [ ] Rain [ ] Cloudy [ ] Snow [ ] Fog [ ] Hazy	[ ] Calm (waves less than 6") [ ] Choppy (waves 6" - 2') [ ] Rough (waves 2' - 6') [ ] Very Rough (greater than 6') [ ] Strong Current	Air _____ °F Water _____ °F	[ ] None [ ] Light (0-6 mph) [ ] Moderate (7-14 mph) [ ] Strong (15-25 mph) [ ] Storm (over 25 mph)	Day Night [ ] Good [ ] [ ] Fair [ ] [ ] Poor [ ]

NAME OF OPERATOR	OPERATOR ADDRESS		
OPERATOR TELEPHONE NUMBER ( ) [ ] Male [ ] Female	DATE OF BIRTH mo day yr	OPERATOR'S EXPERIENCE [ ] Under 10 hours [ ] 10 - 100 hours [ ] Over 100 hours	FORMAL INSTRUCTION IN BOATING SAFETY [ ] State Course [ ] U.S. Power Squadron [ ] USCG Auxiliary [ ] American Red Cross [ ] Informal [ ] None
NAME OF OWNER	OWNER ADDRESS		
OWNER TELEPHONE NUMBER ( )	NUMBER OF People on Board	NUMBER OF People Being Towed	RENTED BOAT? [ ] Yes [ ] No

BOAT NO. 1 (This vessel)

BOAT REGISTRATION OR DOCUMENTATION NUMBER	STATE	HULL IDENIFICATION NUMBER	BOAT NAME
BOAT MANUFACTURER	MODEL	LENGTH	YEAR BUILT

TYPE OF BOAT	HULL MATERIAL	ENGINE	PROPULSION	PERSONAL FLOTATION DEVICES (PFDs)
[ ] Open Motorboat [ ] Cabin Motorboat [ ] Auxiliary Sail [ ] Sail (only) [ ] Rowboat [ ] Canoe/Kayak [ ] Personal Watercraft [ ] Pontoon Boat [ ] Houseboat [ ] Other (specify)	[ ] Wood [ ] Aluminum [ ] Steel [ ] Fiberglass [ ] Rubber/vinyl/canvas [ ] Rigid Hull Inflatable [ ] Other (specify)	[ ] Outboard [ ] Inboard [ ] Inboard- Sterndrive (I/O) [ ] Airboat FUEL [ ] Gasoline [ ] Diesel [ ] Electric	[ ] Propeller [ ] Water Jet [ ] Air Thrust [ ] Manual [ ] Sail NO. OF ENGINES TOTAL HORSEPOWER	Was the boat adequately equipped with COAST GUARD APPROVED PFDs? [ ] Yes [ ] No Were PFDs accessible? [ ] Yes [ ] No FIRE EXTINGUISHERS On Board [ ] Yes [ ] No Used [ ] Yes [ ] No [ ] N/A

OPERATION AT TIME OF ACCIDENT (check all applicable)	ACTIVITY AT TIME OF ACCIDENT (check all applicable)	TYPE OF ACCIDENT	WHAT CONTRIBUTED TO ACCIDENT (check all applicable)
[ ] Cruising [ ] Changing Direction [ ] Changing Speed [ ] Drifting [ ] Towing [ ] Being Towed [ ] Rowing/Paddling [ ] Sailing [ ] Launching [ ] Docking/Undocking [ ] At Anchor [ ] Tied to Dock/Moored [ ] Other (specify)	[ ] Fishing [ ] Tournament [ ] Hunting [ ] Swimming/Diving [ ] Making Repairs [ ] Waterskiing/Tubing/Etc. [ ] Racing [ ] Whitewater Sports [ ] Fueling [ ] Non-Recreational [ ] Other (specify)	[ ] Grounding [ ] Capsizing [ ] Flooding/Swamping [ ] Sinking [ ] Fire or Explosion (Fuel) [ ] Fire or Explosion (Other than Fuel) [ ] Skier Mishap [ ] Collision with Vessel [ ] Collision with Fixed Object [ ] Collision with Floating Object [ ] Falls Overboard [ ] Falls in Boat [ ] Struck by Boat [ ] Struck by Motor/Propeller [ ] Other [ ] Hit and Run	[ ] Weather [ ] Excessive Speed [ ] No Skier Lookout [ ] Restricted Vision [ ] Overloading [ ] Improper Loading [ ] Hazardous Waters [ ] Alcohol Use [ ] Drug Use [ ] Hull Failure [ ] Machinery Failure [ ] Equipment Failure [ ] Operator Inexperience [ ] Operator Inattention [ ] Congested Waters [ ] Passenger/Skier Behavior [ ] Dam/Lock [ ] Other (specify)

ESTIMATED SPEED
[ ] Under 10 mph   [ ] 10 - 20 mph   [ ] Over 20 mph   [ ] Over 40 mph

*Source: USCG Auxiliary, *Boating Safely Instructor's Manual*, 1997.

APPENDIX E *Accident Report Form*

	DECEASED (If more than 2 fatalities, attach additional forms)			
NAME OF VICTIM	ADDRESS OF VICTIM			
DATE OF BIRTH [ ] Male [ ] Female	DEATH CAUSED BY	[ ] Drowning [ ] Other		[ ] Disappearance
	WAS PFD WORN?	[ ] Yes [ ] No		
NAME OF VICTIM	ADDRESS OF VICTIM			
DATE OF BIRTH [ ] Male [ ] Female	DEATH CAUSED BY	[ ] Drowning [ ] Other		[ ] Disappearance
	WAS PFD WORN?	[ ] Yes [ ] No		
	INJURED (If more than 2 injuries, attach additional form)			
NAME OF VICTIM	ADDRESS OF VICTIM			
DATE OF BIRTH	MEDICAL TREATMENT BEYOND FIRST AID?		[ ] Yes	[ ] No
	ADMITTED TO HOSPITAL?		[ ] Yes	[ ] No
	DESCRIBE INJURY			
	WAS PFD WORN? [ ] Yes [ ] No	PRIOR TO ACCIDENT?	[ ] Yes	[ ] No
	WAS IT INFLATABLE? [ ] Yes [ ] No	AS A RESULT OF ACCIDENT?	[ ] Yes	[ ] No
NAME OF VICTIM	ADDRESS OF VICTIM			
DATE OF BIRTH	MEDICAL TREATMENT BEYOND FIRST AID?		[ ] Yes	[ ] No
	ADMITTED TO HOSPITAL?		[ ] Yes	[ ] No
	DESCRIBE INJURY			
	WAS PFD WORN? [ ] Yes [ ] No	PRIOR TO ACCIDENT?	[ ] Yes	[ ] No
	WAS IT INFLATABLE? [ ] Yes [ ] No	AS A RESULT OF ACCIDENT?	[ ] Yes	[ ] No
	OTHER PEOPLE ABOARD THIS BOAT (If more than 2 people, attach additional form)			
NAME	ADDRESS			
DATE OF BIRTH	WAS PFD WORN? [ ] Yes [ ] No	PRIOR TO ACCIDENT?	[ ] Yes	[ ] No
	WAS IT INFLATABLE? [ ] Yes [ ] No	AS A RESULT OF ACCIDENT?	[ ] Yes	[ ] No
NAME	ADDRESS			
DATE OF BIRTH	WAS PFD WORN? [ ] Yes [ ] No	PRIOR TO ACCIDENT?	[ ] Yes	[ ] No
	WAS IT INFLATABLE? [ ] Yes [ ] No	AS A RESULT OF ACCIDENT?	[ ] Yes	[ ] No
	VESSEL NO. 2 (If more than 2 vessels, attach additional form)			
NAME OF OPERATOR	OPERATOR ADDRESS			
OPERATOR TELEPHONE NUMBER	BOAT REGISTRATION OR DOCUMENTATION NUMBER		STATE	
NAME OF OPERATOR	OPERATOR ADDRESS			
OPERATOR TELEPHONE NUMBER	BOAT REGISTRATION OR DOCUMENTATION NUMBER		STATE	
	PROPERTY DAMAGE			
NAME OF OWNER OF DAMAGED PROPERTY OTHER THAN VESSELS	ADDRESS			
ESTIMATED AMOUNT THIS BOAT $ OTHER BOAT(s) $ OTHER PROPERTY $	DESCRIBE PROPERTY DAMAGE			

APPENDIX E *Accident Report Form*

ACCIDENT DESCRIPTION

DESCRIBE WHAT HAPPENED (Sequence of events. Include Failure of Equipment. If diagram needed, attach seperately. Continue on additional sheets if necessary. Include any information regarding the involvement of alcohol and/or drugs in causing or contributing to the accident. Including any descriptive information about the use of PFDs.)

WITNESSES NOT ON THIS VESSEL

NAME	ADDRESS	TELEPHONE NUMBER ( )
NAME	ADDRESS	TELEPHONE NUMBER ( )
NAME	ADDRESS	TELEPHONE NUMBER ( )

PERSON COMPLETING REPORT

NAME	ADDRESS	TELEPHONE NUMBER ( )
SIGNATURE	QUALIFICATION [ ] Operator [ ] Owner [ ] Investigator [ ] Other	DATE SUBMITTED

(Do not use) FOR REPORTING AUTHORITY REVIEW (Use agency date stamp)

Causes based on (check one) [ ] This report [ ] Investigation and this report [ ] Investigation [ ] Could not be determined	Name of Reviewing Officer	Date Received

Appendix F: State Boating Law Administrators*

(Alphabetical by State)

Director, Marine Police Division
Department of Conservation and Natural Resources
674 North Union Street, Room 756
Montgomery, Alabama 36130
Tel. (205)242-3673-3676
Fax. (205)240-3336

Assistant Commander
Department of Public Safety
Pago Pago, American Samoa 96799
Tel. (684)633-1111
Fax. (684)633-7035

State Boating Administrator
Arizona Game and Fish Department
2222 West Greenway Road
Phoenix, Arizona 85023
Tel. (602)942-3000/ext. 491
Fax. (602)789-3920/1

Boating Safety Program Administrator
Arkansas Game and Fish Commission
#2 Natural Resources Drive
Little Rock, Arkansas 72205
Tel. (501)223-6399
Fax. (501)223-6447

Director
Department of Boating and Waterways
1629 S Street
Sacramento, California 95814
Tel. (916)445-9657
Fax. (916)327-7250

Boating Administrator
Division of Parks and Outdoor Recreation
13787 South Highway 80
Littleton, Colorado 80125
Tel. (303)791-1954
Fax. (303)470-0782

Boating Law Administrator
DEP Complex
PO Box 271
163 Great Hill Road
Portland, Connecticut 06480
Tel. (203)344-2668
Fax. (203)344-2560

Boating Law Administrator
Division of Fish and Wildlife
Richardson & Robbins Building
PO Box 1401
Dover, Delaware 19903
Tel. (302)739-3440
Fax. (302)739-3491

Metropolitan Police Department
MPDC Harbor Branch
550 Water Street, SW
Washington, DC 20024
Tel. (202)727-4582
Fax. (202)727-3663

Boating Law Administrator
Florida Marine Patrol
3900 Commonwealth Boulevard
Tallahassee, Florida 32399-3000
Tel. (904)488-5757
Fax. (904)488-6425

Department of Natural Resources
Assistant Chief, Law Enforcement
2109-A U.S. Highway 278, S.E.
Social Circle, Georgia 30279
Tel. (404)656-3534/3510
Fax. (404)656-4992

---

*Source: USCG Auxiliary, *Boating Safely Instructor's Manual*, 1997.

APPENDIX F State Boating Law Administrators

Boating Law Administrator
Guam Police Department
Special Programs Section
287 West O'Brien Drive
Agana, Guam 96910
Tel. (671)472-8911
Fax. (671)472-9704

State Boating Manager
Department of Transportation
79 South Nimitz Highway
Honolulu, Hawaii 96813
Tel. (808)548-2838/2515
Fax. (808)587-1977

Boating Program Supervisor
Department of Parks and Recreation
PO Box 83720
Boise, Idaho 83720-0065
Tel. (208)334-4199
Fax. (208)334-3741

Boating Law Administrator
Division of Law Enforcement
Department of Conservation
524 South Second Street
Springfield, Illinois 62701-1787
Tel. (217)782-6431
Fax. (217)785-8405

State Boating Law Administrator
Department of Natural Resources
402 W Washington Street, Room W-255D
Indianapolis, Indiana 46204
Tel. (317)232-4010
Fax. (317)232-8035

Director, Department of Natural Resources
Wallace Building
Des Moines, Iowa 50319-0035
Tel. (515)281-8688
Fax. (515)281-8895

Boating Administrator
Kansas Wildlife and Parks
RR2, Box 54A
Pratt, Kansas 67124
Tel. (316)672-5911/ext. 158
Fax. (316)672-6020

Director, Kentucky Water Patrol
Department of Natural Resources
107 Mero Street
Frankfort, Kentucky 40601
Tel. (502)564-3074
Fax. (502)564-6193

Boating Law Administrator
Department of Wildlife and Fisheries
PO Box 98000
Baton Rouge, Louisiana 70898-9000
Tel. (504)765-2988
Fax. (504)765-2832

Inland Fisheries and Wildlife
284 State Street, Station #41
Augusta, Maine 04333
Tel. (207)289-2766
Fax. (207)289-6395

Maryland Department of Natural Resources
Tawes State Office Building
580 Taylor Avenue
Annapolis, Maryland 21401
Tel. (301)974-3548
Fax. (301)974-2740

Director
Division of Law Enforcement
100 Nashua Street
Boston, Massachusetts 02114
Tel. (617)727-3905
Fax. (617)727-2754

Chief, Law Enforcement Division
Department of Natural Resources
PO Box 30028
Lansing, Michigan 48909
Tel. (517)373-1230
Fax. (517)373-6186

Boat and Water Safety Coordinator
Department of Natural Resources
Box 46, 500 Lafayette Road
St. Paul, Minnesota 55155-4046
Tel. (612)296-3310
Fax. (612)296-0902

Boating Law Administrator
Department of Wildlife, Fisheries and Parks
PO Box 451
Jackson, Mississippi 39205
Tel. (601)364-2187
Fax. (601)364-2125

Commissioner, Missouri State Water Patrol
Department of Public Safety
PO Box 1368
Jefferson City, Missouri 65102-1368
Tel. (314)751-3333
Fax. (314)636-8428

APPENDIX F *State Boating Law Administrators*

Boating Law Administrator
Boating Safety Division
Department of Fish, Wildlife and Parks
1420 East 6th Avenue
Helena, Montana 59620
Tel. (406)444-2452
Fax. (406)444-4952

Boating Law Administrator
Game and Parks Commission
PO Box 30370
Lincoln, Nebraska 68503-0370
Tel. (402)471-5579
Fax. (402)471-5528

Chief, Division of Law Enforcement
Department of Wildlife
PO Box 10678
Reno, Nevada 89520-0022
Tel. (702)688-1500
Fax. (702)688-1595

Director of Administration
New Hampshire Department of Safety
Hazen Drive
Concord, New Hampshire 03305
Tel. (603)271-2589
Fax. (603)271-3903

Boating Law Administrator
New Jersey State Police
Marine Law Enforcement Bureau
PO Box 7068
West Trenton, New Jersey 08628-0068
Tel. (609)882-2000/ext. 2530/2531
Fax. (609)882-6523

Boating Administrator
Energy, Minerals and Natural Resources Department
Parks and Recreation Division
PO Box 1147
Santa Fe, New Mexico 87504-1147
Tel. (505)827-3986
Fax. (505)827-4001

Director, Bureau of Marine and Recreational Vehicles
Agency Building #1, 13th Floor
Empire State Plaza
Albany, New York 12238
Tel. (518)474-0445
Fax. (518)474-4492

Executive Director
Wildlife Resource Commission
512 North Salisbury Street
Archdale Building
Raleigh, North Carolina 27604-1188
Tel. (919)733-3391
Fax. (919)733-7083

Boat and Water Safety Coordinator
State Game and Fish Department
100 North Bismarck Expressway
Bismarck, North Dakota 58501-5095
Tel. (701)221-6300
Fax. (701)221-6832

Chief, Division of Watercraft
Department of Natural Resources
Fountain Square, C-2
Columbus, Ohio 43224
Tel. (614)265-6480
Fax. (614)267-8883

Director, Lake Patrol Division
Department of Public Safety
PO Box 11415
Oklahoma City, Oklahoma 73136-0415
Tel. (405)425-2143
Fax. (405)425-2268

Director
State Marine Board
435 Commercial Street, N.E.
Salem, Oregon 97310
Tel. (503)378-8587
Fax. (503)378-4597

Director, Bureau of Boating
Pennsylvania Fish and Boat Commission
PO Box 1673
Harrisburg, Pennsylvania 17105-1673
Tel. (717)657-4538
Fax. (717)657-4549

Commissioner of Navigation
Department of Natural Resources
PO Box 5887
Puerta de Tierra, Puerto Rico 00906
Tel. (809)724-2340
Fax. (809)724-7335

Division of Enforcement
Department of Environmental Management
83 Park Street
Providence, Rhode Island 02903-1037
Tel. (401)277-3070
Fax. (401)277-6823

APPENDIX F *State Boating Law Administrators*

Boating Law Administrator
Wildlife and Marine Resources Department
PO Box 12559
Charleston, South Carolina 29412
Tel. (803)762-5041
Fax. (803)762-5007/5001

Boating Safety Coordinator
Department of Game, Fish and Parks
Anderson Building, 445 East Capitol
Pierre, South Dakota 57501
Tel. (605)773-4506
Fax. (605)773-6245

Supervisor, Water Safety Law Enforcement
Texas Parks and Wildlife Department
4200 Smith School Road
Austin, Texas 78744
Tel. (512)389-4850
Fax. (512)389-4740

Boating Law Administrator
Tennessee Wildlife Resources Agency
PO Box 40747
Nashville, Tennessee 37204-9979
Tel. (615)781-6682
Fax. (615)741-4606

Boating Law Administrator
Division of Parks and Recreation
1636 West North Temple Street
Salt Lake City, Utah 84116
Tel. (801)538-7341
Fax. (801)538-7315

Boating Law Administrator
Vermont State Police Headquarters
103 South Main Street
Waterbury, Vermont 05676
Tel. (802)244-8778
Fax. (802)244-1106

Boating Law Administrator
Department of Planning and Natural Resources
Nisky Center, Suite 231
St. Thomas, Virgin Islands 00802
Tel. (809)774-3320
Fax. (809)775-5706

Boating Law Administrator
Department of Game and Inland Fisheries
PO Box 11104
Richmond, Virginia 23230-1104
Tel. (804)367-1189
Fax. (804)367-9147

Boating Safety Administrator
Washington State Parks and Recreation Commission
7150 Cleanwater Lane (KY-11)
Olympia, Washington 98504
Tel. (206)586-2165
Fax. (206)753-1594

Chief, Law Enforcement Section
Division of Natural Resources
Capitol Complex Boulevard East
1900 Kanawha Boulevard East
Charleston, West Virginia 25305
Tel. (304)558-2784
Fax. (304)348-2768

Boating Law Administrator
Department of Natural Resources
PO Box 7924
Madison, Wisconsin 53707
Tel. (608)266-0859
Fax. (608)267-3579/266-3696

Wildlife Law Enforcement Coordinator
Game and Fish Department
5400 Bishop Boulevard
Cheyenne, Wyoming 82006
Tel. (307)777-4579
Fax. (307)777-4610

Director
Department of Public Safety
Civic Center
Saipan, CNMI 96950
Tel. (670)234-6021/606
Fax. (670)234-2023

References

American Camping Association. *Camp Boating Program and Curriculum Guidelines.* Martinsville, IN: American Camping Association, 1993.

American Camping Association. "Camp Boating Survey Summary." American Camping Association, 1994.

American Camping Association. *Standards for Day and Resident Camps.* Martinsville, IN: American Camping Association, 1993.

American Canoe Association. *Canoeing and Kayaking.* Birmingham: Menasha Ridge Press, 1987.

American Canoe Association. *River Safety Anthology.* Walbridge, C., and Tinsley J. Birmingham: Menasha Ridge Press, 1996.

American Canoe Association. *River Safety Report.* Walbridge, C. Birmingham: Menasha Ridge Press, 1996.

The American National Red Cross. "American Red Cross National Boating Survey." Washington, D.C.: 1991.

The American National Red Cross. *CPR for the Professional Rescuer.* St. Louis: Mosby, 1993.

_____. *Basic Water Safety.* Washington D.C.: The American Red Cross, 1988.

_____. *Community Water Safety.* St. Louis: Mosby, 1995.

_____. *Head Lifeguard.* St. Louis: Mosby, 1995.

_____. *Lifeguarding Today.* St. Louis: Mosby, 1995.

_____. *Responding to Emergencies,* ed 2. St. Louis: Mosby, 1995.

_____. *Sport Safety Training: Injury Prevention and Care Handbook.* St. Louis: Mosby, 1997.

_____ . *Canoeing.* Washington, D.C.: The American National Red Cross, 1977.

_____ . *Canoeing and Kayaking.* Washington, D.C.: The American National Red Cross, 1981.

Auerbach, P.S. *Wilderness Medicine.* St. Louis: Mosby, 1995.

Bechdel, L.; and Ray, S. *River Rescue,* 3rd ed. Boston: Appalachian Mountain Club Books, 1997.

Canadian Red Cross Society. *Swimming and Water Safety.* St. Louis: Mosby, 1995.

CCA Safety Committee. *"A Profile of Whitewater Fatalities (1975 through 1991)."* CCA Safety Committee, Revision 5/12/93.

Girl Scouts of the U.S.A. *Safety Wise.* New York, N. Y.: Girl Scouts of the U.S.A., 1993.

Gordon, I. H. *Canoeing Made Easy,* Old Saybrook, Connecticut: The Globe Pequot Press, 1992.

National Safety Council. *Accident Facts 1996 Edition.* Itasca, IL: 1996.

Rescue 3 International. *Swiftwater Rescue Technician I.* Segerstrom, Croslin, Edwards. Elk Grove, CA: Rescue 3, 1997.

Smith & Smith, *Water Rescue.* St. Louis: Mosby, 1994.

Stuhaug, D. *Kayaking Made Easy,* Old Saybrook, Connecticut: The Globe Pequot Press, 1995.

United States Coast Guard, "Boating Statistics 1994," Washington D.C., September 1995.

U.S. Coast Guard Auxiliary. *Boating Safely.* St. Louis: Mosby, 1997.

U.S. Coast Guard Auxiliary. *Skipper's Safe Boating Course,* St. Louis: Mosby, 1996.

United States Marine Corps. "Marine Combat Instructor Water Survival," Camp Lejeune, North Carolina.

U.S. Sailing, *Start Sailing Right,* Portsmouth, RI: United States Sailing Association, 1997.

Walbridge, C.; and Sundmacher, W. A. Sr. *Whitewater Rescue Manual,* Camden, Maine: Ragged Mountain Press.

Index

A
Abdominal thrusts, emergency care and, 34
Accident report form, 8
Accidents
 boating; *see* Boating accidents
 sailing, prevention of, 54-56
Active drowning victim, 27
 definition of, 22
Activity, hypothermia and, 33
Aerial flares, nighttime visual distress signals and, 8
Age, hypothermia and, 33
Air
 in pants in self-rescue, 24
 in shirt or jacket in self-rescue, 23-24
Air bags in kayak, 47, 48
Alcohol, 5
American Canoe Association, 39, 40, 48
American Red Cross Small Craft Safety course, 2
American Whitewater Affiliation (AWA), 40, 48, 70
Ankle sprains
 canoeing safety and, 40
 kayaking safety and, 48
Aquatic emergencies; *see* Emergencies
Assist
 reaching; *see* Reaching assist
 team wading, 74, 75
 throw bag, with belay, 74, 75
 throwing; *see* Throwing assist
 towing; *see* Towing assist
 wading, 30
 walking, 30, 31
Assisting others in flat water
 canoeing emergencies and, 41-43
 kayaking emergencies and, 50
AWA; *see* American Whitewater Affiliation

B
Back blows, emergency care and, 34-35
Back injuries, 31-32
 canoeing safety and, 40
 kayaking safety and, 48
Basic water rescue; *see* Water rescue, basic
Beach drag, 30, 31
Beam, 8
Belay, throw bag assist with, moving-water emergencies and, 74
Bells, sound devices and, 8
Boat
 chase, definition of, 62
 decked, 4
 safety; *see* Safety boat
Boating accident report, 8
Boating accidents
 prevention of, 4-7
 reporting of, legal requirements and, 8
Body size, hypothermia and, 33
Boom of sailboat, 54
Boots, 15
Bow
 of canoe, 39
 of kayak, 47
 of rowboat, 63
 of sailboat, 54
Breathing, rescue, 31, 34
Broach pin, entrapment in canoe or kayak and, 73
Buoyant cushions, 5
Buoyant vests, 5
Buoys, ring, 5, 29

C
Canoe trip leader, canoeing safety and, 40
Canoeing emergencies, 40-43
 assisting others in flat water, 41-43
 canoe-over-canoe rescue and, 43
 falls overboard in flat water, 41
 in flat water, 40-43
 moving water and; *see* Moving-water emergencies
 rescue priorities in, 40
 self-rescue in flat water, 40-41
 swamped canoe in flat water, 41, 42
 towing assist and, 41, 43
Canoeing safety, 38-45
 communication and, 40
 emergencies and; *see* Canoeing emergencies
 guidelines for, 40
 helmets and, 14
 moving water and, 69-77
 prevention of capsizes, collisions, and falls overboard in, 40
 rules of the road and, 7
 supervision and, 40
Canoe-over-canoe rescue, 43
Canoes, 2, 3
 characteristics of, 39
 definition of, 1
 entrapment in, moving-water emergencies and, 73, 74
 outfitting, 40
 swamped, in flat water, 41, 42
Capacity plate, 8
Capalene clothing, 15
Capsize recovery method for one sailor, sailing emergencies and, 58, 59
Capsizes, 5, 6-7
 canoe, prevention of, 40
 definition of, 1
 kayak, prevention of, 48
 in moving water, 71-72
 prevention of, 6-7
 rowboat
  prevention of, 64
  self-rescue from, 64, 65

100

Index

sailing
    prevention of, 56
    self-rescue after, 58
Care, standard of, 12
    definition of, 11
Centerboard of sailboat, 54
Centerboard sailboats, self-rescuing, 58
Chase boat
    definition of, 62
    leader location and, 15
Chest thrusts, emergency care and, 35
CISD; see Critical incident stress debriefing
Closed craft, 47
Clothing
    choice of, in trip planning, 15
    self-rescue with, 23-24, 25, 26
Coaming of kayak, 47
Cockpit of kayak, 4, 47
Cold water, 3
    hypothermia and, 32-34
    predicted survival in, 33
Collisions, 5
    canoe, prevention of, 40
    definition of, 1
    prevention of, 7
    sailing, prevention of, 54-56
Communication
    canoeing safety and, 40
    emergency action plan and, 17
    kayaking safety and, 48
    moving-water safety and, 70-71
    sailing safety and, 57, 58
    small craft supervision and, 15
Core temperature, hypothermia and, 33
CPR, 34, 35
Crew overboard shout, sailing safety and, 59
Critical incident stress
    definition of, 11
    following emergency, 17-19
Critical incident stress debriefing (CISD) following emergency, 19
Critical Incident Stress Foundation, 19
Current
    river, 3
    velocity of, force of water and, 71
Cushions, buoyant, 5

D

Daggerboards of sailboat, 54
Dams, low-head; see Low-head dams
Debriefing, critical incident stress, following emergency, 19
Deck of kayak, 47
Decked craft, 4, 47
Delayed-help situation, 17
Depressions, moving-water emergencies and, 72
Distress lights, nighttime visual distress signals and, 8
Distressed swimmer, 27
    definition of, 22
Drag, beach, 30, 31
Drowning, 4, 5
    definition of, 1
    rowboat safety and, 63
Drowning victim
    active, 27
        definition of, 22
    passive, 27
        definition of, 22
Dry suit, 15

E

EAP; see Emergency action plan
Eddy
    definition of, 69
    moving water emergencies and, 71
Electric torches, nighttime travel and, 8
Emergencies
    canoeing; see Canoeing emergencies
    kayaking; see Kayaking emergencies
    moving water; see Moving-water emergencies
    preparation for, 15-19
    recognizing, 26-27
    sailing; see Sailing emergencies
Emergency action plan (EAP), 19
    contents of, 16-17
    definition of, 11
    in emergency preparation, 16-17
Emergency care, 31-35
    for head, neck, and back injuries, 31-32
    for hypothermia, 32-34
    for seizures, 34
    for unconscious victim, 34
Emergency Medical Services (EMS) personnel, definition of, 22
Emergency Medical Services (EMS), 34
    definition of, 11
    emergency action plan and, 16
Emergency preparation, 15-19
    critical incident stress and, 17-19
    critical incident stress debriefing and, 19
    emergency action plan in, 16-17
    follow-up of, 17-19
    reports and, 17
    trip planning and supervision and, 11-21
Emergency telephone calls, 18
EMS system; see Emergency Medical Services
Entrapment
    in canoe or kayak, moving-water emergencies and, 73, 74
    definition of, 69
    foot; see Foot entrapment
Environment, layout of, emergency action plan and, 16
Equipment
    choice of, in trip planning, 14
    emergency action plan and, 16
    group items of, 14
    personal items of, 14
    reaching assist with, 27
    reaching assist without, 28
    safety, 14
    wading assist with, 30
Exit, wet; see Wet exit
Exposure, length of, hypothermia and, 33

F

Facility, layout of, emergency action plan and, 16
Falls overboard, 5, 6-7
    definition of, 1
    in flat water, canoeing emergencies and, 41
    in moving water, 71-72
    prevention of, 6-7
        canoe, 40
        rowboat safety and, 64
        sailboat safety and, 56
    self-rescue from, rowing emergencies and, 64, 65
Fatalities
    prevention of, 4-7
    rowing, 63-64
    sailing, 54-56

Federal boating laws, accident reporting and, 8
Flares
  aerial, 8
  handheld, 8
Flashlights, nighttime travel and, 8
Flat water
  assisting others in
    canoeing emergencies and, 41-43
    kayaking emergencies and, 50
  canoeing emergencies in, 40-43
  definition of, 38
  falls overboard in, canoeing emergencies and, 41
  kayaking emergencies in, 48-50
  self-rescue in
    canoeing emergencies and, 40-41
    kayaking emergencies and, 48, 49
  swamped canoe in, 41, 42
  wet exit in, kayaking emergencies and, 48, 49
Flat-bottom rowboats, 4, 63
Float plan, 12
  definition of, 11
Floating
  self-rescue and, 23
  survival, self-rescue and, 23
Flooding in rivers and streams, 3
Flotation vests, 5
Follow-up
  after emergency, 17-19
  emergency action plan and, 17
Foot entrapment
  definition of, 69
  moving-water emergencies and, 73
Force of water, current velocity and, 71

G
Gender, hypothermia and, 33
Grab loop of kayak, 47, 48
Group items of equipment in trip planning, 14
Group leader, selection of, in trip planning, 12
Gunwale, 6
  of canoe, 39
  of rowboat, 63
  of sailboat, 54

H
Hand signals
  moving-water safety and, 70
  sailboat safety and, 57, 58
Handheld flares, nighttime visual distress signals and, 8
Hat, 15, 25
Head, neck, and back injuries
  emergency care for, 31-32
  stabilizing, using head splint, 31, 32
  stabilizing, using hip/shoulder support, 32
Head splint, stabilizing head, neck, and back injuries using, 31, 32
Heart rhythms, rapid rewarming and, 34
Heat Escape Lessening Posture (HELP) position, self-rescue when wearing a life jacket and, 25, 26
Heaving jug, 28
Heaving line, 28-29
Heel
  definition of, 53
  sailboats and, 56
Heimlich maneuver, emergency care and, 34
Helmets, 14, 70
HELP position; see Heat Escape Lessening Posture
Hip/shoulder support, stabilizing head, neck, and back injuries using, 32
Holes
  definition of, 69
  moving-water emergencies and, 72
Horns, sound devices and, 8
Huddle position, self-rescue when wearing a life jacket and, 26
Hull
  of canoe, 39
  of rowboat, 63
  of sailboat, 54
Hybrid inflatable personal flotation device, 5, 6
Hydraulics, 3
  definition of, 69
  moving-water emergencies and, 72
Hypothermia
  definition of, 22
  emergency care for, 32-34
  prevention of, 34

I
Incident report form, 18
Inflatable kayaks, 4
Inflatable personal flotation devices, 5, 6
Injuries
  back; see Back injuries
  head, neck, and back, emergency care for, 31-32
  prevention of, 4-7
  rowing, prevention of, 63-64
  sailing, prevention of, 54-56
  shoulder; see Shoulder injuries

J
Jacket, air in, in self-rescue, 23-24
Jibe
  definition of, 53
  of sailboat, 56

K
Kapok, ring buoys and, 29
Kayaking emergencies, 48-50
  assisting others in flat water, 50
  in flat water, 48-50
  kayak-over-kayak rescue in, 50
  moving water and; see Moving-water emergencies
  rescue priorities and, 48
  self-rescue in flat water, 48, 49
  towing assist and, 50
  wet exit in flat water, 48, 49
Kayaking safety, 46-52
  communication and, 48
  emergencies and; see Kayaking emergencies
  guidelines for, 48
  helmets and, 14
  moving water and, 69-77
  rules of the road and, 7
  supervision and, 48
Kayak-over-kayak rescue, kayaking emergencies and, 50
Kayaks, 2, 4
  characteristics of, 47
  definition of, 1
  entrapment in, moving-water emergencies and, 73, 74
Keel of sailboat, 56

L
Lakes, water safety on, 2
Lanterns, nighttime travel and, 8

Lawsuits, 12
Lead craft, leader location and, 15
Leader
   canoe trip, canoeing safety and, 40
   selection of, in trip planning, 12
Leader location in small craft supervision, 15
Leader-to-participant ratios in small craft supervision, 15
Leeward sailboat, right of way of, 54, 56
Legal requirements, 7-8, 12
Length of exposure, hypothermia and, 33
Liability, 12
   definition of, 11
Life jackets; see Personal flotation devices (PFDs)
Lifeguard training, 2, 27
Lightning, 13
Lightning safe position, 13
Lights
   distress, nighttime visual distress signals and, 8
   navigation, legal requirements and, 8
Locale, selection of, in trip planning, 12
Low-head dams, 3
   definition of, 69
   moving-water emergencies and, 72, 73

M

Main sheet of sailboat, 54
Marine law authorities, accident reporting and, 8
Mast of sailboat, 54
Moving water
   canoeing and kayaking safety and, 69-77
   communication on, 70-71
   guidelines for safety in, 70
   power of, 71
   safety and, 69-77
   supervision on, 70-71
Moving-water emergencies, 71-74
   capsizes and, 71-72
   entrapment in canoe or kayak and, 73, 74
   falls overboard and, 71-72
   foot entrapment and, 73
   holes and, 72
   hydraulics and, 72
   low-head dams and, 72, 73
   rescuing others in, 74
   self-rescue in, 71-73
   strainers and, 73
   team wading assist in, 74, 75
   throw bag assist with belay in, 74, 75
Murkiness of water in lakes and ponds, 2

N

National Oceanic and Atmospheric Administration (NOAA), 13
Navigation lights, legal requirements and, 8
Navigation Rules: International-Inland, 56
Neck injuries; see Head, neck, and back injuries
Negligence, 12
Nighttime travel, navigation lights and, 8
Nighttime visual distress signals, 8
9-1-1 systems, 18
NOAA; see National Oceanic and Atmospheric Administration

O

Oars of rowboat, 63
Oceans, water safety on, 3
Open water
   definition of, 1
   water safety in, 2-3
Overboard, falls; see Falls overboard
Overboard recovery, sailing emergencies and, 59-60

P

Paddle suit, 15
Painter of canoe, 39
Pants, air in, in self-rescue, 24, 25, 26
Participant-to-leader ratios in small craft supervision, 15
Passive drowning victim, 27
   definition of, 22
Personal flotation devices (PFDs), 2, 5-6
   canoeing safety and, 39
   damaged, 6
   definition of, 1
   hybrid inflatable, 5
   hypothermia and, 33, 34
   inflatable, 5, 6
   legal requirements and, 8
   self-rescue with, 25-26
Personal items in trip planning, 14
PFDs; see Personal flotation devices
Physical fitness level, hypothermia and, 33
Pinned craft, retrieving, 74
Planning, trip; see Trip planning
Polypropylene clothing, 15
Ponds, water safety on, 2
Port, sailboats and, 54
Port tack, 55
   definition of, 53
Portages, 12, 14
Post-traumatic stress disorder, 19

R

Rapid rewarming, hypothermia and, 34
Reaching assist
   with equipment, 27
   without equipment, 28
   rowing emergencies and, 64, 66
Registration, small craft, legal requirements and, 7
Removal from water in basic water rescue, 30, 31
Reports following emergency, 17
Rescue, 26-30
   canoeing emergencies and, 40
   canoe-over-canoe, 43
   kayaking emergencies and, 48
   kayak-over-kayak, 50
   moving-water emergencies and, 74, 75
   rowing emergencies and, 64-66
   sailing emergencies and, 58
Rescue breathing, 31, 34
Responsibilities
   emergency action plan and, 17
   in trip planning, 12
Rewarming, rapid, hypothermia and, 34
Rigging
   definition of, 53
   of sailboat, 58
Ring buoys, 5, 29
River currents, 3
Rivers, water safety on, 3
Rocker
   definition of, 62
   of rowboat, 63
Route, selection of, in trip planning, 12
Rowboats, 2, 4
   characteristics of, 63
   definition of, 1
   flat-bottom, 4, 63

Index

Rowing accidents, prevention of, 63-64
Rowing emergencies, 64-66
    reaching assist in, 64, 66
    rescue priorities in, 64
    rescuing others from water, 64-66
    self-rescue in, 64, 65
Rowing safety, 62-68
    emergencies and; see Rowing emergencies
    guidelines for, 64
    preventing accidents, injuries, and fatalities in, 63-64
    rules of the road and, 7
Rudder of sailboat, 54
Rules of the road
    definition of, 1
    in preventing collisions, 7

S

Safe shelters, lightning and, 13
Safety
    canoeing; see Canoeing safety
    kayaking; see Kayaking safety
    rowboat; see Rowing safety
    sailing; see Sailing safety
    small craft; see Small craft safety
Safety boat
    definition of, 62
    leader location and, 15
Safety equipment, choice of, in trip planning, 14
Safety position
    definition of, 53
    of sailboat, 50
Sailboats, 2, 4
    characteristics of, 54, 55
    definition of, 1
    leeward, right-of-way of, 54, 56
    righting, after capsize, 58
    windward, right-of-way of, 54, 56
Sailing capsizes, self-rescue after, 58
Sailing emergencies, 58-60
    capsize recovery method for one sailor in, 58, 59
    overboard recovery in, 59-60
    prevention of, 54-56
    rescue priorities in, 58
    scoop recovery method in, 58, 59
    self-rescue after sailboat capsize in, 58, 59
Sailing safety, 53-61
    communication in, 57, 58
    emergencies and; see Sailing emergencies
    preventing capsizes in, 56
    preventing collisions in, 54-56
    preventing falls overboard in, 56
    preventing fatalities in, 54-56
    preventing injuries in, 54-56
    preventing sailing accidents in, 54-56
    rules of the road and, 7
    supervision in, 57, 58
Scoop recovery method, sailing emergencies and, 58, 59
Sea kayaks, 4
Seizures, 23
    emergency care for, 34
Self-rescue, 23-26
    after sailboat capsize, 58, 59
    from capsized or swamped rowboat, 64, 65
    from falls overboard, rowing emergencies and, 64, 65
    in flat water
        canoeing emergencies and, 40-41
        kayaking emergencies and, 48, 49
    HELP position in, 25, 26
    huddle position in, 26
    in moving water, 71-73
    rowing emergencies and, 64, 65
    survival floating and, 23
    when fully clothed, 23-24, 25, 26
    when wearing a life jacket, 25-26
Self-rescuing sailboats, 58
Shelters, safe, lightning and, 13
Shepherd's crook, reaching assist and, 27
Shirt, air in, in self-rescue, 23-24
Shoes, 15, 23
Shoulder injuries
    canoeing safety and, 40
    kayaking safety and, 48
Signals
    hand; see Hand signals
    kayaking safety and, 48
    visual distress, legal requirements and, 8
Sit-on-top kayaks, 4
Small craft, definition of, 2
Small craft capacity, legal requirements and, 8
Small craft registration, legal requirements and, 7
Small craft safety, 1-10
    basic water rescue and, 22-37
    canoeing safety and; see Canoeing safety
    emergency preparation and, 11-21
    kayaking safety and; see Kayaking safety on lakes, 2
    legal requirements in, 7-8
    in moving water, 69-77
    on the ocean, 3
    in open-water environments, 2-3
    on ponds, 2
    preventing accidents, injuries, and fatalities in, 4-7
    on rivers, 3
    rowboat safety and; see Rowing safety
    sailboats and; see Sailing safety
    on streams, 3
    supervision and, 11-21
    trip planning and, 11-21
    types of small craft and, 3-4
    water safety guidelines and, 2
Sound devices, legal requirements and, 8
Splint, head, stabilizing head, neck, and back injuries using, 31, 32
Sprains, ankle; see Ankle sprains
Spray skirt of kayak, 48
Staff responsibilities, emergency action plan and, 17
Standard of care, 12
    definition of, 11
Starboard, sailboats and, 54
Starboard tack, 54, 55
    definition of, 53
State boating administrator, accident reporting and, 8
State boating laws, accident reporting and, 8
Stern
    of canoe, 39
    of kayak, 47
    of rowboat, 63
    of sailboat, 54
Stern seat of rowboat, 63
Strainers, 3
    definition of, 69
    moving-water emergencies and, 73
Streams, water safety on, 3
Stress, critical incident, 17-19
    definition of, 11
Supervision, 15
    canoeing safety and, 40

kayaking safety and, 48
leader location and, 15
leader-to-participant ratios and, 15
moving-water safety and, 70-71
sailing safety and, 57, 58
small craft, 15
trip planning and emergency preparation and, 11-21
Support personnel, emergency action plan and, 16
Survival floating, self-rescue and, 23
Swamped canoe in flat water, 41, 42
Swamped rowboat, rowing emergencies and, 64, 65
Sweep craft, leader location and, 15
Swimmer, distressed, 27
definition of, 22
Swimming, self-rescue and, 23

T

Tack
definition of, 53
port, 55
starboard, 54, 55
definition of, 53
Tandem, paddling, canoeing safety and, 40
Tandem kayaks, 4
Team wading assist, moving-water emergencies and, 74, 75
Telephone calls, emergency, 18
Temperature
core, hypothermia and, 33
water, hypothermia and, 33
Thigh straps, 14, 70
Throw bag, 28, 29
Throw bag assist with belay, moving-water emergencies and, 74, 75
Throwable devices, 5
Throwing assist, 28-29
rowing emergencies and, 64-66
Thunder, 13
Thunderstorm warning, 13
Thunderstorm watch, 13
Thwarts of canoe, 39
Tiller of sailboat, 54

Torches, electric, nighttime travel and, 8
Towing assist
canoeing emergencies and, 41, 43
kayaking emergencies and, 50
Trails, portage, 12, 14
Transom of rowboat, 63
Treading water, self-rescue and, 23
Trim, 6
definition of, 1
Trip planning, 12-15
checking craft and equipment in, 14
clothing choices in, 15
equipment choices in, 14
leader selection in, 12
locale selection in, 12
responsibilities and legal considerations in, 12
route selection in, 12
safety equipment in, 14
supervision and emergency preparation and, 11-21
water conditions in, 13-14
weather conditions in, 12-13

U

Unconscious victim, emergency care for, 34
Universal River Signals, American Whitewater Affiliation, 70

V

Vertical pin, entrapment in canoe or kayak and, 73
Vests; see also Personal flotation devices
buoyant, 5
flotation, 5
Victim
active drowning, 27
definition of, 22
passive drowning, 27
definition of, 22
unconscious, emergency care for, 34
Visual distress signals, legal requirements and, 8

W

Wading assist with equipment, 30

Walking assist, 30, 31
Warm water
floating facedown in, 23
self-rescue in, 23-24
Water
cold; see Cold water
condition of, in trip planning, 13-14
flat; see Flat water
force of, current velocity and, 71
moving; see Moving water
open; see Open water
removal from, in basic water rescue, 30, 31
warm; see Warm water
Water rescue, basic, 22-37
beach drag in, 30, 31
emergency care in; see Emergency care
guidelines for, 27
reaching assist with equipment in, 27
reaching assist without equipment in, 28
recognizing aquatic emergencies in, 26-27
removal from water in, 30, 31
self-rescue; see Self-rescue
throwing assist in, 28-29
wading assist with equipment in, 30
walking assist in, 30, 31
Water safety guidelines, 2
Water temperature, hypothermia and, 33
Weather conditions in trip planning, 12-13
Wet exit
definition of, 46
in flat water, kayaking emergencies and, 48, 49
Wet suit, 15
Whistles
moving-water safety and, 70
sound devices and, 8
White-water kayaks, 4
Windward sailboat, right-of-way of, 54, 56
Wool clothing, 15

MISSION OF THE AMERICAN RED CROSS

The American Red Cross, a humanitarian organization led by volunteers and guided by its Congressional Charter and the Fundamental Principles of the International Red Cross Movement, will provide relief to victims of disaster and help people prevent, prepare for, and respond to emergencies.

ABOUT THE AMERICAN RED CROSS

To support the mission of the American Red Cross, nearly 1.5 million paid and volunteer staff serve in some 1,750 chapters and blood centers throughout the United States and its territories and on military installations around the world. Supported by the resources of a national organization, they form the largest volunteer service and educational force in the nation. They help people prevent, prepare for, and cope with emergencies, whether those emergencies involve blood, disasters, tissue transplants, social services, or health and safety.

The American Red Cross provides consistent, reliable education and training in injury and illness prevention and emergency care, providing training to nearly 16 million people each year in first aid, CPR, swimming, water safety, and HIV/AIDS education.

All of these essential services are made possible by the voluntary services, blood and tissue donations, and financial support of the American people.

FUNDAMENTAL PRINCIPLES OF THE INTERNATIONAL RED CROSS AND RED CRESCENT MOVEMENT

HUMANITY

IMPARTIALITY

NEUTRALITY

INDEPENDENCE

VOLUNTARY SERVICE

UNITY

UNIVERSALITY